Psychological Treatment for
Patients With
Chronic Pain

Clinical Health Psychology Series

Psychological Treatment for
Patients With
Chronic Pain

BETH D. DARNALL

CLINICAL HEALTH PSYCHOLOGY SERIES

ELLEN A. DORNELAS, Series Editor

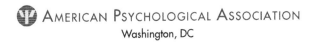
AMERICAN PSYCHOLOGICAL ASSOCIATION
Washington, DC

Published by
American Psychological Association
750 First Street, NE
Washington, DC 20002
www.apa.org

APA Order Department
P.O. Box 92984
Washington, DC 20090-2984
Phone: (800) 374-2721; Direct: (202) 336-5510
Fax: (202) 336-5502; TDD/TTY: (202) 336-6123
Online: http://www.apa.org/pubs/books
E-mail: order@apa.org

In the U.K., Europe, Africa, and the Middle East, copies may be ordered from
Eurospan Group
c/o Turpin Distribution
Pegasus Drive
Stratton Business Park
Biggleswade, Bedfordshire
SG18 8TQ United Kingdom
Phone: +44 (0) 1767 604972
Fax: +44 (0) 1767 601640
Online: https://www.eurospanbookstore.com/apa
E-mail: eurospan@turpin-distribution.com

Typeset in Minion by Circle Graphics, Inc., Columbia, MD

Printer: Sheridan Books, Chelsea, MI
Cover Designer: Mercury Publishing Services, Inc., Rockville, MD

Library of Congress Cataloging-in-Publication Data

Names: Darnall, Beth D., author.
Title: Psychological treatment for patients with chronic pain / by Beth D. Darnall.
Other titles: Clinical health psychology series.
Description: First edition. | Washington, DC : American Psychological Association, [2019] | Series: Clinical health psychology series | Includes bibliographical references and index.
Identifiers: LCCN 2018003705| ISBN 9781433829420 | ISBN 1433829428
Subjects: | MESH: Chronic Pain—psychology | Chronic Pain—therapy | Psychotherapy—methods | Pain Management—psychology | Pain Management—methods
Classification: LCC RB127 | NLM WL 704.6 | DDC 616/.0472—dc23
LC record available at https://lccn.loc.gov/2018003705

British Library Cataloguing-in-Publication Data
A CIP record is available from the British Library.

Printed in the United States of America
First Edition

http://dx.doi.org/10.1037/0000104-000

10 9 8 7 6 5 4 3 2 1

I respectfully dedicate this book to the legends in the fields of pain, psychology, and behavioral pain medicine, whose groundbreaking research procured evidence-based treatment for pain and the material for this book. In writing this book, I endeavored to honor your collective wisdom and transformative work.

Contents

Series Foreword

Mental health practitioners working in medicine represent the vanguard of psychological practice. As scientific discovery and advancement in medicine has rapidly evolved in recent decades, it has been a challenge for clinical health psychology practice to keep pace.

In a fast-changing field, and with a paucity of practice-based research, classroom models of health psychology practice often do not translate well to clinical care. All too often, health psychologists work in silos, with little appreciation of how advancement in one area might inform another. The goal of the Clinical Health Psychology Series is to change these trends and provide a comprehensive yet concise overview of the essential elements of clinical practice in specific areas of health care. The future of 21st-century health psychology depends on the ability of new practitioners to be innovative and to generalize their knowledge across domains. To this end, the series focuses on a variety of topics and provides both a foundation as well as specific clinical examples for mental health professionals who are new to the field.

Working with Susan Reynolds, senior acquisitions editor at the American Psychological Association (APA Books), I am proud to have had an opportunity to edit this book series. We have chosen authors who are recognized experts in the field and who are rethinking the practice of health psychology to be aligned with modern drivers of health care such as population health, cost of care, quality of care, and customer experience.

Dr. Beth D. Darnall is a nationally recognized expert in the psychological treatment of chronic pain. Health psychologists working in both primary care and specialty care areas of medicine routinely encounter medical patients with chronic pain and problematic use of opioid medications. Practitioners who are not expert in pain treatment feel ill prepared to address the needs of their patients with persistent pain. Yet referral to specialty pain clinics is often neither practical nor appropriate. Dr. Darnall guides the mental health professional reader through the complex subject matter of pain treatment, providing a current, state-of-the-science overview, practical resources, illustrative case examples, and a summary of key take-away points. An accompanying video from the APA (*Cognitive Behavioral Therapy for Chronic Pain*; http://www.apa.org/pubs/videos/) features Dr. Darnall demonstrating her approach to pain treatment. *Psychological Treatment for Patients With Chronic Pain* is a wonderful addition to the Clinical Health Psychology Series and will be a complement and frequently used resource in the library of any practicing mental health professional.

—Ellen A. Dornelas, PhD
Series Editor

Foreword

In the wake of the epidemic of problems associated with the escalation of opioid prescribing for pain in the United States, there is an increased awareness of the prevalence and burden of chronic pain as well as interest in effective nonopioid therapies. For the millions of Americans on long-term opioid therapy with questionable benefits and substantial risks, there is an urgent need for treatments to help them effectively manage their pain while tapering off opioids. Cognitive and behavioral approaches are of particular interest given their demonstrated effectiveness and low risk. Unfortunately, this interest and need come at a time when few multidisciplinary pain treatment programs remain and few psychologists with specialized training in pain are available. One of the most frequent complaints I encounter when speaking with primary care physicians is, "Cognitive behavioral therapy is great, and I would love to refer my patients for it, but there is no psychologist anywhere near who does this." There is a great need for more and better education about pain and the effectiveness and risks of various treatments for pain problems; this holds true for physicians, psychologists, other health care professionals, patients, policymakers, and the public. In recognition of the importance of pain education, the International Association for the Study of Pain declared 2018 as the Global Year for Excellence in Pain Education.

Beth D. Darnall draws from her extensive experiences working with individuals with chronic pain problems, in-depth knowledge of evidence-based psychological therapies, and experience working with agencies seeking to improve pain care to write a book that is solidly grounded in evidence yet accessible and practical. This volume provides a comprehensive and up-to-date overview of key concepts important in understanding chronic pain (and the patients living with it), evidence-based psychological therapies for chronic pain, and issues involved in opioid therapy for chronic pain. Readers will also be rewarded with information on useful resources for mental health professionals and their patients. It is my hope that many more psychologists will become involved in helping individuals with chronic pain improve their skills for managing their pain; resolve comorbid problems such as depression, anxiety, and insomnia; and engage in the activities they find pleasurable and meaningful. This is work that can be challenging but also incredibly interesting and rewarding. This book provides a solid foundation for that venture!

—Judith A. Turner, PhD
Professor, Department of Psychiatry & Behavioral Sciences
and Department of Rehabilitation Medicine
Adjunct Professor, Department of Anesthesiology
& Pain Medicine
University of Washington School of Medicine
Seattle, WA

Preface

Welcome to *Psychological Treatment for Patients With Chronic Pain*, a book in the Clinical Health Psychology Series published by the American Psychological Association. This book provides psychologists, trainees, and other health care professionals with information on the critical role of psychology in the experience of pain and its treatment. Knowledge on pain psychology and treatment is bedrock for the clinical health psychologist. After all, pain is the most common health complaint and reason people seek medical care for a variety of health reasons (Schappert & Rechtsteiner, 2008), and chronic pain is the most common chronic health condition in the United States. As you will learn, pain psychology is not just about helping patients cope with pain; rather, pain psychology treatment can reduce pain intensity, alter the trajectory of pain, improve the outcomes of medical treatments, and help patients with pain live more functional and meaningful lives.

A little bit of background about me and how I came to be a pain psychologist. I am a clinical professor in the Department of Anesthesiology, Perioperative and Pain Management at Stanford University School of Medicine. I received my doctorate degree in clinical psychology from the University of Colorado at Boulder. My doctoral studies included zero training in pain, as is commonly the case in graduate clinical psychology programs in the United States. However, I was fortunate to receive my clinical internship training at the Tucson Veterans Affairs (VA) Hospital, where I learned about chronic pain and how to best treat it. I recall starting my internship and working with veterans who had severe chronic pain. I wondered how I could possibly help with their physical pain—it triggered a sense of helplessness in me that is not uncommon to many mental health professionals who lack training in pain. Feelings of helplessness or discomfort about chronic pain are simply information that knowledge and skills are needed. You will learn, as I did, that there is much you can do to alleviate the suffering associated with physical pain.

After my Tucson VA internship I did a postdoctoral fellowship at the Johns Hopkins University School of Medicine in the Department of Physical Medicine and Rehabilitation and in the Bloomberg School of Public Health, where I received advanced pain training in severe medical conditions. At Hopkins, I treated patients after amputation, severe spinal cord injury, and catastrophic burn—conditions that typically involved intense pain, major life adjustment, and psychological distress.

I have been treating patients with pain for 15 years, mainly in academic pain clinics at Oregon Health & Science University and at the Stanford University School of Medicine in California. My work in the field extends beyond patient care to leadership, education, research, and authorship to have a broader impact on chronic pain treatment across multiple disciplines of health care. My past pain leadership roles include serving as the 2012 president of the Pain Society of Oregon and as cochair of the Pain Psychology Task Force at the American Academy of Pain Medicine. I am current cochair of the Behavioral Medicine Committee at the American Academy of Pain Medicine, and also serve on their Opioid Advisory Committee. I have coauthored or advised on the development of national pain treatment guidelines and resources for the American Pain Society (2016), the American College of Occupational and Environmental Medicine (2017), and the American Chronic Pain Association (2015, 2017).

As principal investigator for nationally funded pain research, I work with colleagues to investigate psychological treatments for chronic pain and their ability to reduce the use of prescription opioids and to prevent postsurgical pain (National Institutes of Health, Patient-Centered Outcomes Research Institute). Outside of Stanford, I develop pain psychology treatment programs for major health care systems and consult with agencies and groups wishing to create a clinical cultural transformation in the treatment of pain by integrating pain psychology treatment into primary care and specialty pain clinics. My consulting and national advocacy work have centered on education and training about pain psychology and advancing the presence of psychology in the field of pain medicine and health care in general.

A main focus of my clinical work (and research) involves helping patients reduce their need for and use of opioids. Historically speaking, many patients were prescribed opioids without being offered any alternatives. Often patients received no formal assessment of their psychological history or status prior to prescription—and therefore received no treatment for the psychological factors that were serving to amplify their pain and need for pain medication. I worked with patients who had been taking opioids for months or years who told me that opioids reduced their pain by only a small amount, though the side effects and consequences were large. People were coming to me seeking to learn ways to manage pain without opioid medication or at least less of it. Over and over I was giving the same information to patients one at a time—a highly inefficient process! To meet demand and reach a wider audience, I wrote two patient books (which are also appropriate for mental health professionals): *Less Pain, Fewer Pills: Avoid the Dangers of Prescription Opioids and Gain Control Over Chronic Pain* (2014) and *The Opioid-Free Pain Relief Kit: 10 Simple Steps to Ease Your Pain* (2016). Both books emphasize the role of psychology in the experience of pain and teach people what they can do to reduce their own pain and distress and how psychological skills can be used to reduce need and use of risky pain medications. In 2018, the patient workbook of the Chronic Pain Self-Management Program, an international treatment program, included a chapter that I authored on opioid reduction. In terms of professional education, I coauthored the seventh edition of the American Pain Society book *Principles of Analgesic Use* (2016).

LIVING A HEALTHY LIFE WITH CHRONIC PAIN

My public and mental health professional education efforts include a blog on pain psychology at *Psychology Today*. My research and public education continue to emphasize psychobehavioral treatment as a low-risk, evidence-based pain treatment pathway to reduce need for pain medication.

To help shore the gap for mental health professional and clinician training needs for psychological approaches to chronic pain treatment, I have delivered workshops on behavioral medicine for chronic pain for health care providers (physicians, psychologists, and other clinicians) in national and international venues, including the American Academy of Pain Medicine, the Institute for Brain Potential, and the Israeli Pain Association. Nationally, there is great need and desire to better understand psychological influence on pain and to develop systems that integrate evidence-based psychological treatments for pain into medical care pathways. The risk and side effect profile for psychological treatment pales in comparison to most pharmaceutical, medical, and surgical procedures. And psychological treatment can be as effective as many pain medications or procedures—sometimes more so. The interest in this space extends beyond national borders. In 2018 I presented on The Psychology of Pain Relief at the World Economic Forum in Davos, Switzerland, and my invited commentary on the need to integrate psychology into pain research and treatment was published in the international journal *Nature*.

Helping individuals with chronic pain learn to alleviate their suffering is deeply gratifying work. A common stigma about people with pain is that they are "difficult patients" or "hard to treat." Broadly speaking, in many ways health care has failed people living with chronic pain. Numerous barriers prevent people from accessing the evidence-based, comprehensive pain care that they need. Paradoxically, patients may receive a lot of pain treatments and medical care, just not necessarily ones that are effective or right for them. Clinicians may label patients as difficult when treatment after treatment fails to improve their pain, and understandably patient distress increases.

PAMELA'S EXAMPLE OF HAVING PAIN OVERTREATED AND UNDERTREATED AT THE SAME TIME[1]

Pamela is a 50-year-old woman with chronic low back pain. For the past 5 years she has received about 30 epidural steroid injections a year for her back pain—a lot of medical treatment. Pamela is not working. She has

---

[1]This and all other case examples used throughout the book are fictitious or have been disguised to protect confidentiality.

underlying posttraumatic stress disorder and fear-avoidance behaviors, is deconditioned, and spends most of her day on the sofa or in bed. Some days she does not even get out of bed and get dressed for the day. Although Pamela is getting lots of shots and some pills for her pain, her psychosocial factors have never been assessed or treated. As a result, she remains distressed and feels trapped by her pain, unable to move forward with her life and toward the goals that are meaningful to her.

Pamela is an example of a common paradoxical phenomenon in which pain is overtreated and undertreated at the same time. Her pain is being undertreated because she is not receiving the type of pain care she truly needs. The key to best pain treatment is ensuring that a patient's pain is being treated in the way that is right for them. Almost always, the best pain care involves a comprehensive approach with careful attention to the patient's psychological needs.

I wrote this book to begin to address a gap created by the confluence of four important factors: (a) the striking prevalence of chronic pain, (b) the overlap between chronic pain and mental health factors and problems, (c) the emphasis of the biomedical treatment for pain yielding suboptimal outcomes and contributing to further patient suffering, and (d) a lack of psychologists and mental health professionals who are trained to effectively address pain in the therapeutic context with evidence-based strategies.

Acknowledgments

My heartfelt thanks to the American Psychological Association for prioritizing pain in this Clinical Health Psychology Series and bringing forward this information to mental health and other health care professionals and their current and future patients. My thanks to Ming-Chih Kao, PhD, MD, for providing graphical illustrations of pain and its impacts; to Heather Poupore-King, PhD; to Nita Bryant, Jesmin Asika Ram, and Wendy Schadle for support; to the expert reviewers who contributed helpful recommendations for refinement; and to Erin O'Brien and Joe Albrecht for skillful editing. Finally, I gratefully acknowledge you, the reader, and your dedication to learning about pain and evidence-based pain management strategies. Thank you for becoming empowered to help alleviate the suffering of others.

Psychological Treatment for
Patients With
Chronic Pain

Introduction

The overall goal of this book is to provide you with a high-level over-view of pain psychology and evidence-based psychological treat-ment for pain. The book also includes a clinical tool kit of resources and a road map for further learning about pain psychology. At the end of each chapter, you will find practical resources that you can use with your patients who have pain. Each chapter also contains a bulleted summary of key points and case vignettes that illustrate key concepts and treatment approaches. Collated resources are located at the end of the book, includ-ing multimedia recommendations for further learning, mental health professional clinical tools, and patient resources.

http://dx.doi.org/10.1037/0000104-001
Psychological Treatment for Patients With Chronic Pain, by B. D. Darnall

TERMINOLOGY

The following are different descriptors and labels for commonly used terms, as well as the term selected for this text. Recognizing that there are pros and cons to each choice, the terms chosen were selected for clarity and consistency and to provide the best context within the broad topic.

- Chronic versus persistent pain. *Chronic pain* and *persistent pain* are interchangeable terms. Both are used in this text, with greater use of *chronic*.
- Patients versus clients. If you work outside the medical setting, you are likely to use the term *client* in your practice. For consistency and brevity, the term *patient* is mainly used in this text, particularly in descriptions of medical settings and treatments. It is important to note that advocacy groups such as the American Chronic Pain Association prefer deemphasizing the term *patient* and using a more empowering descriptor, such as "person living with chronic pain."
- Behavioral medicine for pain versus psychobehavioral treatment for pain versus pain psychology. Although these terms are interchangeable, *psychological* or *psychobehavioral* treatment for pain is used more in this text.

THE SCOPE OF THE PROBLEM OF PAIN

Chronic pain is one of the largest health problems worldwide. In the United States, the incidence of chronic pain is greater than diabetes, heart disease, and cancer combined (Institute of Medicine [US] Committee on Advancing Pain Research, Care, and Education, 2011). Chronic pain is the leading cause of disability in the United States and costs the nation $635 billion annually in terms of medical care and lost productivity. At the individual level, chronic pain often confers substantial burdens, limitations, and physical and emotional suffering. Often the negative effects of chronic pain extend beyond the individual to family members, other loved ones, and even coworkers.

About 30% of adults report living with some degree of ongoing pain, and among older adults, the estimate is as high as 40% (Institute of Medicine [US] Committee on Advancing Pain Research, Care, and Education, 2011). Some studies have suggested that more than 10% of the population lives with severe chronic pain. A European survey of individuals with chronic pain found that 90% reported they had been living with chronic pain for more than 2 years, and about one third were receiving no treatment for it (Breivik, Collett, Ventafridda, Cohen, & Gallacher, 2006). It is thought that the high prevalence of chronic pain is partly attributable to the aging of the population and higher obesity rates; research has shown that older age and obesity are associated with a greater likelihood for persistent pain.

The rates of pain in the United States are similar to those reported for population studies in other countries (Institute of Medicine [US] Committee on Advancing Pain Research, Care, and Education, 2011). Regardless of nationality, most people are likely to experience persistent pain at some point in their lives. Chronic pain frequently co-occurs with various psychological symptoms and disorders. As such, it is vitally important for mental health professionals to have a foundational understanding about pain and the role of psychology in the onset, experience, and maintenance of pain and how evidence-based psychological treatments can be used to treat chronic pain and lessen its burdens.

Patients with depression or anxiety often have comorbid acute or chronic pain. If you are a mental health professional, you are likely treating these individuals in your practice. Most psychologists report being ill-equipped to address their patients' chronic pain. Discomfort in treating pain leads to missed opportunities for psychologists to help reduce their clients' suffering. As a mental health professional, you play an important role in the treatment of your patients' pain.

You can avoid the risk of unwittingly reinforcing your patients' maladaptive beliefs and behaviors about pain, thereby fueling cycles of pain and disability. Psychologists need not be pain experts to help current and future patients who have pain. By learning some key basics outlined in this book, you will increase your knowledge and your ability to steer your patients with chronic pain toward effective psychobehavioral treatment.

Often, patients travel far and wide to receive pain care from academic pain clinics because specialized, comprehensive pain services do not exist in many communities and rural areas. Patients tend to receive their pain treatment locally—often at their primary care doctor's office. Increasingly, primary care is evolving toward integrated models that have psychological services embedded in the clinic. However, such progressive integrated primary care is not yet the norm. In the vast majority of primary care settings, pain is likely to be treated as a biomedical problem, thereby leaving psychosocial factors unidentified, unaddressed, and poorly treated. To their credit, physicians may recognize the need for psychological treatment and recommend it to their patients with chronic pain. And patients may seek a mental health professional in their community to receive psychological "support." However, general counseling and psychological support are distinct from evidence-based psychological treatment for pain. And herein lies the problem.

In the pain clinic, my patients would often have a psychologist or mental health therapist they were regularly seeing for supportive therapy or to address depression; however, their pain was not being addressed at all. This problem is not new. Despite the scientific evidence showing that psychological treatment for pain is effective and often essential, few psychologists and mental health professionals are equipped to treat pain. Part of my role as a pain psychologist is to conduct a full pain psychology evaluation and then give the patient recommendations to implement close to where they live—which may be hundreds of miles away from the Stanford pain clinic. Giving a patient a recommendation to work with a local psychologist skilled in treating pain can be futile advice because of the lack of psychologists with specialized training.

From an anecdotal perspective, pain psychologists and pain physicians are keenly aware of the shortage of pain psychologists—and even general psychologists who have basic competency in treating pain—but no data existed to describe contributing factors and potential solutions. To address this gap in understanding, in 2016 the Pain Psychology Task Force of the American Academy of Pain Medicine published the first study to broadly characterize the needs for pain psychology services in the United States and for pain training among psychologists and mental health therapists (Darnall et al., 2016; note that this is an open-access article).

To conduct this study, we surveyed almost 2,000 individuals across six key stakeholder groups: patients with chronic pain ($n = 1,086$), pain physicians ($n = 203$), primary care physicians and physician assistants ($n = 221$), nurse practitioners ($n = 96$), psychologists and mental health therapists ($n = 323$), and directors of graduate and postgraduate psychology training programs ($n = 62$). The partial results of our psychologist survey appear in Table 1.

Sixty-five percent of psychologists and mental health therapists reported that at least a quarter of their clientele has chronic pain. One third reported that at least half their clientele has chronic pain. And yet, mental health therapists also reported having little or no education and training to treat pain and, unsurprisingly, low confidence in their ability to treat pain. Indeed, almost 90% of U.S. mental health therapists surveyed reported a need for education in the treatment of chronic pain.

> Almost 90% of U.S. psychologists surveyed self-identified a need for education in the psychological treatment for chronic pain.

Our finding of low confidence among mental health therapists is an important point because it suggests that therapists (a) may be avoiding the topic of pain with their clients, (b) are treating pain in the wrong ways or not using evidence-based strategies, or (c) both. All three possibilities reveal an exciting opportunity for psychologists to positively affect the mental and physical health of clients with pain education. The need for better pain education extends beyond mental health professionals. Notably, many physicians are uncomfortable treating chronic pain.

> The *biomedical model* approaches pain as a medical problem that requires an external medical treatment. The *biopsychosocial model* recognizes that best pain care includes psychosocial treatment into an integrated, comprehensive approach that engages the patient in their pain care.

Table 1

Psychologist/Therapist National Survey (*N* = 323)

	%	*n*
1. Do you consider yourself to be a specialist in treating patients with pain?		323
No	70.2	227
Yes	22.6	73
Other	7.2	23
2. Please select from the following options which best characterize the amount of education/training you received in pain psychology prior to licensure.		322
Little or no education/training	36.7	118
Clinical experience	19.9	64
Continuing education (conferences, self-study, etc.)	19.6	63
Predoctoral (academic and/or clinical) and postdoctoral training	19.3	62
Postdoctoral level training only	4.7	15
3. Please select from the following options which best describe your perceived level of comfort and competency in treating individuals with pain.	34.1	110
I treat individuals with pain, but feel less confident in my ability to treat these patients than other areas of general psychology.	34.1	110
I consider myself to be competent, but I would benefit from more training and specialized education.	33.8	109
I do not feel competent and therefore do not treat individuals with pain.	20.7	67
I consider myself to be very competent. This is my specialized area of interest.	11.5	37
4. Approximately what percentage of your patients have pain (acute or chronic)?		320
< 25	35.9	115
25–49	27.8	89
50–74	22.5	72
75–100	13.8	44
If a packaged pain psychology curriculum were available to you at no cost, would you be interested in learning more?		323
Yes	91.0	294
No	7.1	23
Other	1.9	6

Many physicians receive as little as 4 to 11 hours of chronic pain training in medical school (Mezei & Murinson, 2011), hardly sufficient to manage the complexities of chronic pain and all the psychosocial issues that accompany it. As such, physicians may find it easier to practice the biomedical treatment model and simply write a prescription to treat chronic pain. The biomedical approach may seem easier in the short run, but it often yields poor results and can create new problems. The biomedical treatment approach is inadequate because it fails to recognize and address the many psychosocial factors that influence chronic pain and affect pain treatment outcomes. Greater burdens for physicians and patients may unfold over time as medical treatments fail and as patients are exposed to health risks from additional medical treatments such as surgery, opioids, and other pharmaceuticals.

The *biopsychosocial treatment model* for chronic pain recognizes that psychosocial factors strongly influence the degree to which one experiences pain. Evidence-based psychological treatment for pain equips patients to use cognitive, emotional, and behavioral skills to reduce their pain and suffering. Evidence-based psychological strategies are shown to improve function, decrease pain, and reduce psychological distress, thereby empowering patients to live life meaningfully within the context of chronic pain and other medical problems (more on this in Chapter 1).

"Chronic pain is a biopsychosocial condition that often requires integrated, multimodal, and interdisciplinary treatment, all components of which should be evidence-based."

—NIH Interagency Pain Research
Coordinating Committee (2015, p. 3)

An ethical imperative exists for psychologists to understand the basics of psychological treatment for pain so that, at a minimum, clients can be steered toward science-backed materials and to qualified experts. My hope, however, is that you may be inspired to pursue advanced training in pain. The needs of the masses simply outweigh the number of psychologists with expertise in pain. In 2016, the National Pain Strategy (NIH Interagency Pain Research Coordinating Committee, 2015) was published as a road map for transforming pain research, education, and policy in the United States. The National Pain Strategy recommended integration of behavioral and self-management strategies broadly into U.S. pain care, and in 2017 this was extended into the National Pain Research Strategy. As discussed in Chapter 9, the U.S. opioid epidemic has fostered a great interest in nonpharmacological and nonopioid pain treatment options. More than ever, the U.S. health care system is in need of behavioral medicine for pain and skilled psychologists to meet this pressing national need.

In this book, Chapters 1 to 5 discuss the nature of pain and comorbid effects, such as depression and anxiety, and look at a broader scope of pain treatment and provide an overview of the common and distinct components in psychological treatments for pain. This will set the stage for understanding some the main ingredients and how they work. Chapters 6 and 7 cover psychobehavioral treatments with the best scientific evidence for chronic pain: cognitive behavioral therapy, acceptance and commitment therapy, mindfulness-based stress reduction, mindfulness meditation, hypnosis, biofeedback, and chronic pain self-management. Overlap exists between these treatment approaches, and there are key distinctions as well. These chapters are meant to provide an overview of the common and distinct components in psychological treatments for pain and to set the stage for understanding some of the main ingredients and how they work.

KEY POINTS

- Up to one third of individuals are living with ongoing pain.
- Psychologists have reported that two thirds of their clients have pain.
- Almost 40% of psychologists have reported having little or no training in pain.
- About 90% of psychologists have reported a need and desire to learn about the psychological treatment of pain.
- Psychosocial factors strongly contribute to the onset and maintenance of pain.

- Best pain care involves a comprehensive biopsychosocial treatment approach.
- Psychologists are a critical part of the solution to treating pain effectively and with lowest risks.
- The 2016 National Pain Strategy called for the expansion of the biopsychosocial treatment approach for chronic pain and the integration of evidence-based behavioral and self-management strategies into national health care systems.

RESOURCES

The National Pain Strategy:

NIH Interagency Pain Research Coordinating Committee. (2015). *National pain strategy: A comprehensive population health-level strategy for pain.* Retrieved from https://iprcc.nih.gov/sites/default/files/HHSNational_Pain_Strategy_508C.pdf

Federal Pain Research Strategy Overview:

NIH Interagency Pain Research Coordinating Committee. (2017). *Federal pain research strategy overview.* Retrieved from https://iprcc.nih.gov/Federal-Pain-Research-Strategy/Overview

A National Center for Biotechnology Information open access article (https://www.ncbi.nlm.nih.gov/pmc/articles/PMC4758272/):

Darnall, B. D., Scheman, J., Davin, S., Burns, J. W., Murphy, J. L., Wilson, A. C., . . . Mackey, S. (2016). Pain psychology: A global needs assessment and national call to action. *Pain Medicine, 17,* 250–263. http://dx.doi.org/10.1093/pm/pnv095

The scientific and ethical imperative to include psychology in pain research and treatment:

Darnall B. (2018). To treat pain, study people in all their complexity. *Nature, 557,* 7. http://dx.doi.org/10.1038/d41586-018-04994-5

Darnall, B. D., Carr, D. B., & Schatman, M. E. (2017). Pain psychology and the biopsychosocial model of pain treatment: Ethical imperatives and social responsibility. *Pain Medicine, 18,* 1413–1415. http://dx.doi.org/10.1093/pm/pnw166

1

The Role of Psychological Factors in Chronic Pain

Chronic pain may arise from many types of medical diagnoses or problems, such as osteoarthritis, rheumatoid arthritis, irritable bowel disease, prolonged high levels of alcohol consumption, sickle cell disease, and diabetic neuropathy, to name just a few examples. Chronic pain may develop after surgery or injuries, when pain unexpectedly fails to resolve with healing. On average, about 10% of all people who undergo surgery will go on to develop postsurgical chronic pain, though rates vary widely depending on the type of surgery (Macintyre, Scott, Schug, Visser, & Walker, 2010). Some surgeries have much higher rates of post-surgical chronic pain, such as amputation (30%–85%), coronary bypass (30%–50%), and total knee arthroplasty (up to 35%).

Iatrogenic pain is pain that is caused or worsened by medical intervention. For instance, some data have suggested that opioids can increase sensitivity to pain, or *hyperalgesia*, in some people (Roeckel, Le Coz,

http://dx.doi.org/10.1037/0000104-002
Psychological Treatment for Patients With Chronic Pain, by B. D. Darnall

Gavériaux-Ruff, & Simonin, 2016). In this example, taking medications as prescribed may promote pain. In other cases, the medication-taking behavior of the patient can cause or contribute to greater pain. For instance, people taking medication for persistent headache can develop a secondary type of headache called *medication overuse headache* (Tepper, 2017). This could be caused by poor prescribing practices or from patients taking too much medication in the false belief that it will help them gain relief. Worsening pain is often treated with even more medication, thereby underscoring the need for nonpharmacologic strategies that can break the negative cycle of pain caused by the treatments. Other examples of iatrogenic pain include injured nerves and peripheral neuropathy that commonly occurs after cancer patients receive chemotherapy and radiation treatments. Treatments that are necessary for survival can result in lasting pain and substantial burdens for individuals and their families.

Idiopathic pain is pain that begins for no clear medical reason. Unexplained pain can be particularly distressing to individuals who seek a medical diagnosis and validation for their pain. Individuals may feel stigmatized and may even hear from others that because their pain is not medically explained it must be of psychological origin. This binary thinking about medical versus psychological is unhelpful. Psychological treatment can benefit virtually any patient with chronic pain, regardless of the cause of pain or the medical diagnosis. It is important for patients to understand that one type of pain is not more legitimate than any other type. Unfortunately, such misperceptions compound suffering for the individual and may contribute to resistance to psychological treatment for pain.

Regardless of its origin, chronic pain is associated with negative impacts across an array of physical and psychosocial domains, including physical functioning, sleep, mood, emotions, cognition, work, and relationships, to name just a few. Chronic pain is a major cause of disability, financial loss, social withdrawal, and isolation. Depression, anxiety, posttraumatic stress disorder, and other psychological disorders commonly co-occur with chronic pain. People with chronic pain are at increased risk of developing psychological disorders, in part because of the physical and emotional suffering, life changes, and losses that may develop as a consequence of chronic pain.

MARGARET'S UNEXPLAINED PAIN

Margaret had severe abdominal pain that no one could figure out.[1] She went to her doctor, sought a second opinion, and then had work-ups by two different gastrointestinal specialists. One doctor thought it might be irritable bowel disorder, but the others did not. And no one knew why her pain started or what was making it worse. The lack of answers made Margaret feel like her invisible chronic pain was doubly invisible because there was no medical "proof" of it. She worried that people did not believe her, and once she heard a health care staff member mention that stress could be part of her problem. Margaret felt offended because the comment seemed to imply that the problem was "all in her head."

Margaret reluctantly agreed to see a pain psychologist to learn how to "cope with" her pain, if nothing else. She was surprised at how much she learned. She learned that all pain is legitimate, regardless of the diagnosis—and that psychology plays an important role in the experience of all chronic pain. In her weekly sessions, she began focusing less on finding a diagnosis or cure and instead began putting her energy toward figuring out what she could do to better her pain and symptoms, including her physical and psychological distress. She found that she was not just coping better with her pain—she was actually changing her pain because her pain episodes were becoming less intense, less frequent, and less bothersome. She began to feel more in control and stopped worrying so much about the things she could not control, such as the medical cause. She still hoped her doctors would figure it out, but she was no longer willing to sit and wait for it. She had too much living to do for that!

THE ROLE OF PSYCHOLOGY IN THE CYCLE OF PAIN

The pain cycle graphic in Figure 1.1 illustrates how pain that arises from injury or surgery leads to sensitization in the peripheral and central nervous systems. Psychological factors amplify these sensitization

---

[1]All case examples used in this chapter are fictitious or have been disguised to protect confidentiality.

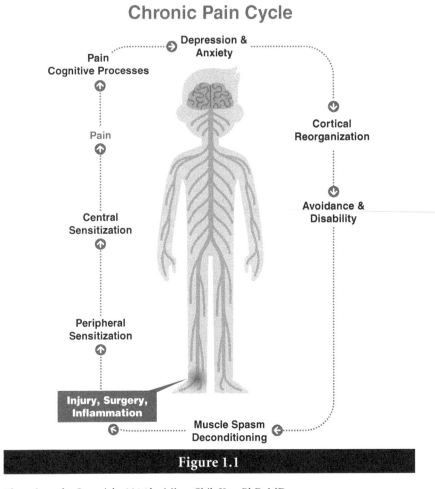

Chronic Pain Cycle

Figure 1.1

The pain cycle. Copyright 2016 by Ming-Chih Kao, PhD, MD.

processes. Such psychological factors may predate the pain, arise in response to the pain, or co-occur. Ongoing distress about pain, anxiety, and depression can contribute to the pain cycle in multiple ways, such as behavior changes and avoidance of activity. Although patients tend to avoid activity in an attempt to reduce or prevent further pain, activity avoidance serves to maintain and worsen the problem over time, as you will learn in Chapter 4.

Psychologists can help patients to break the pain cycle by addressing the psychological and behavioral factors that serve to maintain chronic pain and disability—regardless of how or when they began. Patients will fall along a continuum, anchored on one end by those with poor resources and life-coping skills that predated their pain and on the other end by those with a demonstrated history of resiliency who can adapt to the challenges of chronic pain with some basic education and support. Like other chronic diseases such as diabetes, chronic pain treatment requires lifestyle changes and self-management approaches that help individuals gain control over their pain, increase their functioning, and live better within the context of their medical condition(s). This is best achieved with a comprehensive approach that includes evidence-based physical therapy or movement therapies, medical treatments, psychological approaches (behavioral medicine for pain), and self-management strategies. Evidence-based psychological approaches are essential to effectively address the negative psychological reactions to pain that, left untreated, can complicate the trajectory of pain and amplify suffering. Understanding pain, psychology, and the intersection between the two begins with the definition of pain.

WHAT IS PAIN?

Although pain is often considered to be purely a negative physical sensation, it is much more than just bodily hurt. Psychological factors are integral to the experience and trajectory of pain. As such, psychology is built into the International Association for the Study of Pain (1979) definition of pain as "an unpleasant sensory *and* emotional experience associated with actual or potential tissue damage" (p. 250; italics added).

Despite psychological factors being integral to pain, they are often underappreciated and undertreated. Instead, medical approaches are often emphasized with the biomedical treatment approach. Consequently, pain treatment results and patient outcomes may be limited or poor because major contributing psychosocial factors remain untreated.

> "To consider only the sensory features of pain, and ignore its motivation and affective properties, is to look at only part of the problem, and not even the most important part at that."
>
> —Melzack and Casey (1968, p. 423)

Given the comprehensive definition of pain, it follows that a comprehensive treatment approach is needed. The biopsychosocial treatment model of pain (see Figure 1.2; Gatchel, McGeary, McGeary, & Lippe, 2014) is a more comprehensive approach to treating chronic pain. It discourages a focusing on medical cures, achieving zero pain (both of which are often unrealistic), or waiting for pain to improve before moving forward with one's life. Rather, the biopsychosocial treatment approach encourages patients to become active partners in their pain management and health care. Physicians and medical interventions are just one part of comprehensive pain care plan that includes psychosocial and movement therapies

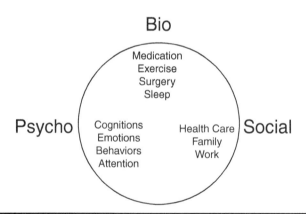

Figure 1.2

The biopsychosocial model of pain emphasizes the dynamic interaction among physiological, psychological, and social factors. Reprinted from "Interdisciplinary Chronic Pain Management: Past, Present, and Future," by R. J. Gatchel, D. D. McGeary, C. A. McGeary, and B. Lippe, 2014, *American Psychologist, 69*, p. 121. Copyright 2014 by the American Psychological Association.

(see Table 1.1), with the patient learning to set realistic functional goals and daily action plans that help improve symptoms, well-being, and self-efficacy and make gradual progress toward the attainment of goals that are meaningful to them.

Psychological factors are integral to the pain experience, and they alter the trajectory of pain by influencing

- response to medical treatments for pain,
- engagement in biopsychosocial treatment for pain (when available), and
- whether patients take an active role in the management of their pain.

Despite decades of research suggesting that biopsychosocial treatment is best, chronic pain is often still treated with the biomedical approach. The reasons why are varied, but as noted in Chapter 1, poor access to pain psychology care remains a major barrier. In addition, few integrated, comprehensive pain treatment centers exist relative to the number of people living with chronic pain. In large part, this is due to the complexities of insurance coverage and poor financial sustainability for many integrated pain clinics or intensive outpatient pain rehabilitation programs. Treating pain comprehensively is more complex and time-consuming than simply writing a prescription, and the current health care system does

Table 1.1	
Where Pain Care Is Received	
General practitioners	Pain specialists
Primary care	Pain clinics
Community practices (e.g., physical therapy, psychology)	Outpatient intensive pain rehabilitation programs
	Functional restoration programs
	Inpatient intensive pain rehabilitation programs (functional restoration programs may also be included here)

not financially reward best care practices. Recent scrutiny of opioid overdose deaths—and the role of prescription opioids in overdose and other health risks—has created fertile ground for the biopsychosocial treatment model to flourish. For instance, the Veterans Affairs (VA) health care system reported that since 2013 the VA has emphasized opioid reduction in veterans taking long-term opioids, thereby leaving a gap for alternative pain treatment approaches. More than ever there is great interest in low-risk, nonopioid treatments (e.g., http://www.usmedicine.com/agencies/department-of-veterans-affairs/as-opioid-prescribing-drops-va-expands-alternative-pain-therapies/). Exciting new evidence supports the efficacy of psychological treatments for pain (Cherkin et al., 2016) as low-risk solutions. Simultaneously, the Internet and social media have helped to broadly disseminate information about best pain care approaches that are low-risk and have lasting results.

MARY'S MIGRAINE PROBLEM AND THE PAIN CYCLE

Mary is a 34-year-old woman who has had headaches since childhood. On a few occasions, she stayed home from school because her head hurt, but they did not affect her functioning much as an adult—until last year. Since then Mary was missing 5 days of work a month because of severe head pain that left her having to lie down in a dark room to gain some relief. She went to her primary care doctor and was diagnosed with migraines. She was given some different pain medicine, but it was not helping much. Her migraines would last for 2 days at a time. When she was having a migraine, she would lie in a dark room and move as little as possible. When her migraine subsided, she would worry about the migraine returning. She felt tense all the time, and her neck ached from the muscle tension. She was avoiding exercise and nonessential movement out of fear that it would cause a new migraine. She stopped going to her walking group and no longer went to the gym with her daughter. The combination of doing less, missing work, and feeling that her life was slipping away was leaving her feeling depressed.

Mary's case illustrates two things: (a) how psychological factors contribute to the pain cycle and (b) how a purely biomedical approach is shortsighted and fails to address the individual factors that may be maintaining and promoting pain and suffering. Like all patients, Mary needs a comprehensive treatment approach that includes assessment and treatment for the psychosocial factors and lifestyle behaviors that are worsening her pain and depression.

Studies show that when major contributing psychological factors are left untreated, medical treatment response may be limited or absent (Archer et al., 2016; Archer, Seebach, Mathis, Riley, & Wegener, 2014; Burns, Glenn, Bruehl, Harden, & Lofland, 2003; Tota-Faucette, Gil, Williams, Keefe, & Goli, 1993; Wertli et al., 2014). Gold-standard pain treatment involves targeting the full definition of pain, including the psychological dimensions. Perhaps a more accurate description of pain is that it is a psychophysical experience, and it stands as an excellent illustration of how mind and body interrelate to affect mental and physical well-being.

MEASURING PAIN

Pain is measured by simply asking a person to rate their pain. Most often a 0- to 10-point scale is used, whereby 0 = *no pain* and 10 = *the most severe pain imaginable*; occasionally a 0-to-100 or a 0-to-5 scale is used. Measuring pain is different from measuring a fixed quantity, such as the volume of water in a glass or using a thermometer to measure the temperature of the air objectively. Pain ratings are not objective; rather, they are highly variable depending on the person, the context, their mood (Carroll, Cassidy, & Côté, 2004) and stress levels (Crettaz et al., 2013), or even the quantity and quality of sleep the night before (Ribeiro-Dasilva, Goodin, & Fillingim, 2012; M. T. Smith & Haythornthwaite, 2004).

Indeed, pain is influenced by many individual factors, such as genetics, race, and sex or gender (Darnall & Suarez, 2009; Fillingim, 2000; Green et al., 2003; see Exhibit 1.1 for a list of factors associated with greater likelihood for persistent pain). For example, African Americans are more likely to

Exhibit 1.1

Factors Associated With Greater Likelihood for Persistent Pain

- History of psychological trauma
- History of abuse
- Lower socioeconomic status
- Female sex
- Age
- Race
- Pain-related anxiety, fear of pain, pain catastrophizing
- Substance use disorder
- Medical comorbidities
- Sleep disorder
- Nutritional status
- Sedentary or low activity levels
- Smoking
- Psychological disorders

Note. For children, additional risks include parental or caregiver history of chronic pain and caregiver psychological distress about their child's pain. See Wilson, Moss, Palermo, and Fales (2014).

experience chronic pain than other races (Campbell & Edwards, 2012). In general, minorities tend to have greater pain, and it is thought that this is caused, in part, by increased stress and poorer health associated with lower socioeconomic status (Brydon, Edwards, Mohamed-Ali, & Steptoe, 2004; Campbell & Edwards, 2012; Carroll, Cassidy, & Côté, 2003). Another example is sex or gender. Although young boys and girls report experiencing the same pain intensity in pain experiments and have about the same incidence of pain conditions, sex or gender differences emerge in adolescence. Among teens, pain is more common and more intense in girls, and coping differences emerge: Girls tend to ruminate more on pain, whereas boys are more likely to use distraction (Lynch, Kashikar-Zuck, Goldschneider, & Jones, 2007). These coping differences persist into adulthood (Unruh,

Ritchie, & Merskey, 1999), with women being more likely to experience chronic pain and to experience greater pain intensity than men (Unruh, 1996). There are many reasons women have more pain than men, including differences in hormones, stress responses, and the immune system (which is one reason women are more likely to have painful conditions such as rheumatoid arthritis, fibromyalgia, and lupus; Bartley & Fillingim, 2013; Bartley et al., 2016; Fillingim, 2015; Tighe, Riley, & Fillingim, 2014). Although women are more sensitive to pain, they are also more likely to seek treatment for it. Women are also more likely to have co-occurring mental health conditions and to seek mental health services.

PAIN AND THE BRAIN: THE BASICS

Understanding the psychology of pain requires basic knowledge of the relationship between pain and the brain. Even though pain is typically perceived as a physical experience, all pain is processed in the brain. If a person sprains his or her ankle, the sensation of pain[2] is felt in that location of the body yet is the product of pain-related information processed in the central nervous system (brain and spinal cord). Pain severity often depends less on medical characteristics and can be more heavily influenced by various personal factors, such as age, sex or gender, genetics, health status, history of trauma or abuse, pain condition, medications, stress, sleep, weight, and psychological status, to name a few (Andreucci, Campbell, & Dunn, 2017; Davis, Luecken, & Zautra, 2005; Fillingim, 2000; Fillingim, King, Ribeiro-Dasilva, Rahim-Williams, & Riley, 2009; Generaal, Vogelzangs, Penninx, & Dekker, 2017; Green et al., 2003; Holbrook, Hoyt, Stein, & Sieber, 2002; see Figure 1.3). Even memories of painful experiences influence subsequent pain (Noel, Chambers, McGrath, Klein, & Stewart, 2012).

A multitude of relevant factors combine to explain why the experience of pain—and pain intensity—varies greatly from one person to the next. On a 0-to-10 pain scale, I may rate my pain intensity a 6, whereas you may rate your pain a 4—much less painful. Pain differences exist even

---

[2]The physical sensation of pain is also referred to as the "sensory experience of pain."

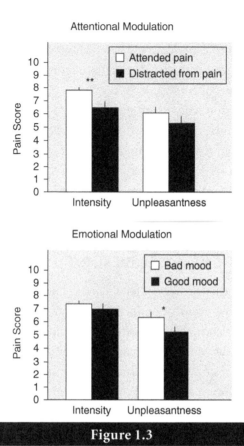

Figure 1.3

Pain is complex. $*p < .05$. $**p < .01$. From "Cognitive and Emotional Control of Pain and Its Disruption in Chronic Pain," by M. C. Bushnell, M. Čeko, and L. A. Low, 2013, *Nature Reviews Neuroscience*, *14*, p. 506. Copyright 2013 by Macmillan Publishers Limited. Reprinted with permission.

when we "standardize" pain in the laboratory to ensure that you and I receive the same degree of heat pain stimulus, for example. We could both have the same 120-degree heat applied to the palms of our hands, and we may experience fairly big differences in the amount of heat pain we feel. As such, there is no standard "sprained ankle" pain score. In the case of a sprained ankle or another injury, it may be tempting to think of pain as being purely a reflection of the severity of the injury. For instance, an 8/10 pain score would reflect a severe sprain, whereas a 3/10 pain score would reflect a milder severity of injury. Although there is some relationship between injury severity and pain intensity score, many times there is only a weak correlation or even no correlation at all (Rosenbloom, Khan, McCartney, & Katz, 2013).

Because pain is processed in the nervous system, anything that affects the nervous system can also affect the experience of pain, regardless of the source of the pain, the type of pain condition one has, results for diagnostic imaging tests, or its etiology.

Psychological factors, such as the context in which pain is felt, one's beliefs about pain, the meaning one attributes to pain, and the amount of attention one gives the pain, influence whether one rates pain from the same stimulus as either higher or lower intensity (Bushnell, Čeko, & Low, 2013). Psychological factors change the experience of pain—for better and for worse. Chapters 3 and 4 cover this content in much greater detail. Regardless of one's medical condition or diagnosis, pain is either amplified or diminished through multiple psychological factors. Such psychological factors become important therapeutic targets for helping patients reduce pain and suffering. Although individuals' medical diagnoses are unlikely to change, their psychological status, how they relate and respond to their pain, and their degree of suffering from pain are highly malleable and serve as the basis for pain psychology treatment.

THE SEARCH FOR A CURE

It is often believed that pain persists because the true medical cause has not been found. Patients may believe that the right diagnosis would lead to proper treatment and resolution of the pain. But it is not always this simple. The search for a diagnosis and cure may involve a multitude of medical tests and imaging, such as X-rays, magnetic resonance imaging (MRI), ultrasound, or computerized axial tomography (CAT or CT) scans. The images are meant to provide meaningful evidence to explain a person's pain, but in fact, images provide limited information about chronic pain. For instance, an analysis of data from multiple studies (meta-analysis) revealed that spine images are weakly correlated with reports of back pain (Brinjikji et al., 2015). Patients may seek confirmation and validation of their pain in images and be left confused and distressed when the cause is not found, leading them to continue to seek medical validation through ongoing testing that may be costly and include health risk exposure (e.g., CT scans). It is important for patients to understand that lack of positive findings for scans or images does not invalidate their experience of pain nor does it imply that their pain has no medical basis.

On the flip side, positive findings for scans or images do not necessarily imply that an individual has pain. A group of researchers sought to reveal the predictive validity of spine-imaging features in asymptomatic populations (Brinjikji et al., 2015). The researchers conducted a meta-analysis by compiling the results of spine-imaging data for more than 3,000 patients taken from 33 different studies of healthy individuals with no back pain. They found that almost 40% of pain-free young adults between 20 and 30 years of age showed evidence of disc degeneration in their spine images. Aging increases the likelihood of having evidence of spine degeneration. Almost all the pain-free individuals 80 years of age or older (96%) had spine degeneration on their images—despite having no pain. The researchers found similar results for spine disc bulges and protrusions (Brinjikji et al., 2015). Patients with degenerative spine image results may despair or catastrophize their imaging results, experience psychological distress, and falsely believe a prognosis of disability when, in fact, their images may hold little explanatory or predictive value.

Mental health professionals can play an important role in helping patients understand the importance of looking beyond medical images, instead helping them to focus more on what they can do to manage pain and increase function. It is understandable for patients to seek diagnostic confirmation and visual validation of their pain because they are living with a "hidden" condition. Many patients with chronic pain experience negative social impacts, such as stigma, disbelief, or misunderstanding from friends, loved ones, or coworkers, thereby fueling the search for validation. Psychologists can help patients understand that it is important to optimize self-management strategies, even as they continue to look for a diagnosis and the right medical treatment. Guiding patients to focus on what they can do to help themselves as early on as possible will facilitate recovery and rehabilitation.

THE UP SIDE OF PAIN: SURVIVAL

Pain is a natural part of life for virtually all humans, and it serves a protective function that promotes survival. A small number of people born with congenital insensitivity to pain, a rare genetic condition, are unable to feel pain. These individuals tend to die young because they lack the crucial internal protective mechanism of pain. They may bite off their tongue and break bones without knowing it; such frequent, severe injuries can have fatal consequences. It is useful to consider the value of pain, its role in human survival, and how it serves as a powerful "harm alarm." The brain registers pain as a danger signal, and it shapes human behavior to move toward relief and physical safety.

> Pain serves as a "harm alarm," a warning signal to urge humans to escape whatever is causing pain and potentially threatening survival.

Consider the pain felt when a person touches a hot stove. Pain will register as a danger signal, and it will strongly motivate quick escape from the "threat"—in this case, the hot stove top—and removal of the hand from the heat. In doing so, further burn and harm are avoided. Or consider a scenario in which a person is walking barefoot and accidentally steps on a sharp tack. The resulting stabbing pain will instantly grab attention, thereby serving as a useful harm alarm, and there will be strong motivation to escape the pain, remove the tack, and protect the foot. The hot stove and sharp tack examples illustrate the responses and utility of short-term, acute pain. The utility and protective value of acute pain diminish over time and can actually contribute to problems for people living with chronic pain. To understand why, let us first review the distinction between short-term pain (acute pain) and longer term pain (chronic or persistent pain).

ACUTE AND CHRONIC PAIN

Acute pain is defined as pain that is limited to less than 3 months in duration and/or occurs during the expected course of healing. In cases of injury, such as a broken ankle, acute pain can help the healing process by serving as an "alarm" to trigger protective behaviors and thereby prevent further tissue damage. The pain will prevent an injured person from vigorous activity and will encourage behavior that will allow for healing. In this sense, acute pain adaptively promotes health and survival.

Chronic pain lasts longer than 3 months or beyond the expected time of healing. For some medical conditions, persistent pain can be a sign of ongoing disease processes (e.g., cancer, pancreatitis). However, in most cases, chronic pain is neither useful nor does it promote healing because the pain persists long after tissue has healed, when no alarm or protection is needed. Even in cases with no clear original injury, such as chronic migraine, the ongoing pain serves no clear useful function. However, some patients may learn—through close listening to their body and its signals—that their pain can serve as a guide to adaptive behavioral change (e.g., activity pacing, improved posture, rest, setting limits with others). Chronic pain is often indirectly related to changes caused by the original incident or disease, including ones that occur in the nervous system's pain detection system (International Association for the Study of Pain, 2018). For this reason, chronic pain is considered a disease in its own right. (See Table 1.2 for a comparison of acute and chronic pain.)

With the exception of congenital pain conditions, all pain begins as acute pain. How and why acute pain may persist and become chronic is a topic of much interest, research, and mystery. Research has shown that various medical and psychosocial factors are associated with the development of chronic pain (transition of pain from the acute to chronic state), as well as ongoing treatment needs. For instance, negative expectations and beliefs about pain or treatment (nocebo responses[3]) have been shown to amplify

---

[3]*Nocebo* is the belief or expectation that a treatment or event will have a negative effect, such as increased pain.

Table 1.2	
Acute Versus Chronic Pain	
Acute pain	Chronic pain
Lasts less than 3 months.	Lasts longer than 3 months.
Usually associated with damage to body tissue.	Persists beyond expected time of healing.
Resolves with healing.	Often has no clear adaptive function.
Serves as a warning signal to protect oneself from further harm.	For some medical conditions it can be a sign of ongoing disease processes (e.g., cancer, pancreatitis). More often, it has little or no protective value.
Examples: burns, broken bones, sprained ankles, sore throats, infections, cuts, procedural dental pain.	Examples: neuropathic pain from cancer treatments received 2 years prior, persistent migraines, total body pain, fibromyalgia, persistent back pain 1 year after surgery.

pain and are linked to hyperalgesia (Colloca & Benedetti, 2007) and findings from neuroimaging research illustrate that negative expectations for pain cause increased pain processing in key brain regions (Bingel et al., 2011).

Psychological factors affecting the duration of pain, fear of pain, pain catastrophizing, and depressive symptoms have all been prospectively associated with pain persistence after acute injury or surgery (Archer et al., 2014; Burton, Tillotson, Main, & Hollis, 1995; Linton, 2005), and some research has suggested psychological factors predict opioid use, including long-term use (Helmerhorst, Vranceanu, Vrahas, Smith, & Ring, 2014; Sun, Darnall, Baker, & Mackey, 2016). Other research has suggested that psychological factors, including beliefs about pain and pain treatment, may mediate or moderate response to opioid analgesia (Bingel et al., 2011), thereby underscoring the imperative to consider and optimize psychological factors and functioning to reduce pain, treatment needs, and negative impacts.

Indeed, chronic pain is associated with an array of negative impacts and burdens to the individual, including sleep disturbance, dependence on medications, dependence on family or caregivers, high medical service use, work-related and functional disability, social isolation, anxiety, fear, anger, depression, and in some cases, suicide. By addressing the psychological and environmental factors that may be maintaining or amplifying pain and suffering (and therefore increasing treatment needs), psychologists play an important role in helping patients mitigate the negative impacts of pain across domains of life and health, thereby helping to restore engagement in meaningful life pursuits and overall quality of life.

Patients with chronic pain naturally wish to understand the cause or source of their pain. Severe and debilitating chronic pain may begin spontaneously or for no known reason, or it may be triggered by a minor injury or event, such as stepping hard off a curb. *Complex regional pain syndrome* (CRPS; also called reflex sympathetic dystrophy; https://www. ninds.nih.gov/Disorders/Patient-Caregiver-Education/Fact-Sheets/ Complex-Regional-Pain-Syndrome-Fact-Sheet) is a condition that results after trauma or injury to a limb. Regardless of whether the trauma was major or minor, the event triggers an abnormal response in the peripheral and central nervous system. In addition to pain, signs and symptoms of CRPS include skin texture changes (the skin becomes shiny and waxy looking), skin color and temperature changes, hair growth pattern changes, nail growth changes, and inflammation. CRPS may behave like an infection and spread to other body parts and limbs. For example, a person could develop CRPS in their thumb after jamming it while catching a baseball. The pain in the thumb could spread to the whole hand and arm, or it may spread to the opposite arm. Although it is often said that chronic pain is invisible and therefore overlooked by the world, CRPS is one of the few pain conditions for which some of the symptoms are visible.

TODD'S STORY OF COMPLEX REGIONAL PAIN SYNDROME

Todd injured his foot in a soccer game at college. It seemed like something that would probably go away in a few days, but he grew concerned when it actually got worse. His foot turned red and felt hot. It felt like it was on fire. He thought if he just protected his foot it would heal. He made an appointment with his doctor, and when the X-rays and other images were normal, he was encouraged to rest for a bit. He started using crutches.

Todd's concern became frank distress. As the weeks and months passed, he found he was still unable to walk on his foot. He tried several different medications, and nothing helped. His foot was still so painful he did not want anyone to touch it, let alone move it. The redness and swelling would come and go, and his toenails were growing strangely. Finally, he was referred to a pain physician who diagnosed him with CRPS. He learned that his care plan would include working with a psychologist and a physical therapist weekly. Together, his therapists helped him to slowly begin moving his foot while also helping him combat his intense fear of using his foot. He was given movement and psychology exercises to practice at home each day, and slowly he increased his ability to move his foot with less fear and distress. It was a slow process, but for the first time, he could imagine a future with no crutches. He set a goal of being crutch free in 3 months.

Todd's story above is an example of chronic pain arising from an injury. Chronic pain may arise from a variety of other medical reasons, such as an illness like shingles. Shingles is caused by herpes zoster, the virus that causes chicken pox. Herpes zoster remains dormant in everyone who has had chicken pox. Later in life—typically around age 50 or so—in some people, the virus becomes active again and develops into shingles, a painful rash that appears on the face or trunk of the body. Although the skin rash heals and disappears, what often remains is chronic nerve pain known as postherpetic neuralgia.

Chronic pain may also be caused by various conditions, such as fibromyalgia or diseases such as Lyme or inflammatory bowel disease.

Unlike acute pain, chronic pain confers no survival value. There is no ongoing, external threat to escape from and therefore no need for a harm alarm. This is the riddle of chronic pain: Humans are wired to want to escape pain, but one cannot simply "escape" chronic pain. As such, chronic pain leads to conscious and unconscious stress in the nervous system (Moseley, Nicholas, & Hodges, 2004) coupled with a host of difficult emotions. But as the false alarm of pain continues to ring, it triggers common changes in the muscles, brain and spinal cord, breathing patterns, heart rate, thoughts, and emotions—changes that can lead to greater pain if they are not addressed.

> Over time, pain loses its protective value as a harm alarm. Once chronic, pain becomes a distressing "false alarm" because there is no threat one can escape. Learning to calm this distressing false alarm is a critical aspect of psychological pain management.

PAIN INTERFERENCE, LOSS OF PHYSICAL FUNCTION, AND DISABILITY

Individuals often say that the worst part of chronic pain is how the pain has interfered with their lives and robbed them of the things they love. Indeed, ongoing pain can cause people to become less active in an attempt to gain relief (so-called fear-avoidance behavior). Fear-avoidance behavior can lead people to do fewer of the activities that are enjoyable and meaningful to them. Participation in recreational and social activities may dwindle, and one can easily become socially withdrawn and isolated. As one's world becomes smaller and smaller, pain and despair may grow and become the primary focus of one's life. It is important to address fear avoidance because it leads to greater disability (Archer et al., 2014; Buer & Linton, 2002; Denison, Asenlöf, & Lindberg, 2004). Doing less and less contributes to the development of depressive symptoms, deconditioning, disability, and—paradoxically—greater pain (Kroska, 2016). A major aspect of effective treatment for chronic pain involves encouraging clients to move beyond their fear of pain and forward again—at an appropriate pace—toward the goals that are meaningful to them and important for their health.

KEY POINTS

- Pain is a brain-based phenomenon; it is a product of the nervous system.
- Pain is personal: Pain intensity varies substantially from person to person, even in situations in which the stimulus is standardized.
- Pain intensity also varies greatly within each person, depending on a multitude of factors, such as the context in which pain is experienced, the meaning attributed to pain, hormone levels, mood, stress, and sleep.

- There can be a weak relationship between injury severity and pain intensity.
- There can be a weak relationship or no relationship between anatomical pathology (imaging results) and pain. Someone with degenerative changes in their spine may have no pain, whereas someone with severe spine pain may have a normal MRI result.
- Psychological disorders and pain frequently co-occur.
- Psychological disorders and pain are bidirectionally related and have shared mechanisms.
- Women are more likely to have chronic pain and psychological disorders and to seek treatment for both.
- Pain is a psychosensory experience (psychology is a component of pain).
- Psychological factors are underappreciated and undertreated in the context of pain.
- Psychologists play a critical role in helping patients understand pain and how they can reduce their suffering.

RESOURCES

A free download on the role of psychologists in managing pain (with contributions from D. Bruns and R. Kerns):

American Psychological Association Help Center. *Managing chronic pain: How psychologists can help with pain management.* Retrieved from http://www.apa.org/helpcenter/pain-management.pdf

Discussion of the neurobiology of the psychological dimensions of chronic pain:

Bushnell, M. C., Čeko, M., & Low, L. A. (2013). Cognitive and emotional control of pain and its disruption in chronic pain. *Nature Reviews Neuroscience, 14,* 502–511. http://dx.doi.org/10.1038/nrn3516

2

Standard Medical Treatments for Pain and Treatment Decision Considerations

This chapter is meant to demystify aspects of the medical world of pain management. Although it is not necessary to become a medical expert, some medical context is helpful for treating patients with pain and likely will expand on your mental health training. This chapter provides some basic information on pain treatment approaches and rationales, as well as medical vocabulary that will allow a degree of foundational knowledge in your patient discussions. Basic information about pain medications can help you appreciate their cognitive and emotional effects.

Medical pain treatment options are generally determined by a patient's specific pain diagnosis. Determining whether a patient is a good candidate for medical treatment requires individual considerations. A health or pain psychologist will conduct an in-person psychological evaluation with the patient and review their current and historical medical and psychosocial factors. Psychologists arrive at a recommendation regarding a patient's

http://dx.doi.org/10.1037/0000104-003
Psychological Treatment for Patients With Chronic Pain, by B. D. Darnall

candidacy for higher risk pain treatments, such as surgical implantation of a spinal cord stimulator, by carefully reviewing the patient's psychosocial factors, history, and the evidence for how those factors affect pain and treatment outcomes. Although the *Diagnostic and Statistical Manual of Mental Disorders* diagnoses are important factors to consider, other factors heavily influence whether a patient is a good candidate for certain medical procedures. Examples of such factors include patients' level of functioning, their response to past medical treatments, whether they have a passive versus active approach to their health and pain care, their current engagement in comprehensive pain treatment, their motivation to engage in evidence-based active self-management, and their past response to medical treatments.

In short, psychosocial factors can preclude candidacy for medical interventions when data suggest that such factors will (a) undermine patients' treatment response, (b) potentially worsen a pain condition, or (c) enable patients to maintain a passive role in their pain care.

DONNA'S STORY

Donna's pain began 15 years ago after a major car accident.[1] At the time, it was mainly spine and neck pain from whiplash and a back injury she sustained in the accident. Donna never returned to work after the accident. Instead, she was homebound, had panic attacks almost daily, and stopped driving her car. She could endure car rides only if she took Valium first. Donna learned early on that movement made her pain worse, so in attempt to reduce her pain she stopped moving much at all. She spent most of her days either in bed on sitting in her house on the Internet or watching TV.

"My doctor prescribed me an opioid medication, Norco, which I take three times a day," Donna said. "I follow the prescription to the letter, but my pain is still so severe I can barely move! I just need better pain control so I can live a normal life and spend time with my grandkids."

---

[1]All case examples used in this chapter are fictitious or have been disguised to protect confidentiality.

Donna's doctor referred her to a specialist who noted that she was a good medical candidate for surgical implantation of an intrathecal pump—a little device that would deliver opioid medication locally, right at the site of her back pain, and reduce her use of oral opioid medication. As such, the pump option would minimize the side effects of oral opioids including severe constipation, poor sleep, and ongoing anxiety she had about getting her prescriptions on time. Donna's doctor referred her for a psychological evaluation to determine whether she was an appropriate candidate for surgical implantation of the morphine pump.

Donna's psychological evaluation included a review of her available medical records that dated back 10 years, an hour-long in-person clinical interview, and multiple psychological tests that she completed on the day of her psychological visit. The full evaluation revealed that Donna had current untreated posttraumatic stress disorder (PTSD), panic disorder with agoraphobia, and severe fear of pain. Her main coping strategy was fear-avoidance behaviors: She was avoiding anything that might increase her pain, and she was also avoiding anything that would increase her anxiety, such as driving. Because she was inactive, she was deconditioned and was relying almost solely on medications to manage her pain. She had no active coping strategies and had avoided physical rehabilitation because of her fear of worsening pain.

From a psychological perspective, Donna was deemed a poor candidate for a morphine pump for the following reasons:

- Untreated PTSD is associated with postsurgical pain, poor recovery, and greater use of opioids.
- Untreated PTSD amplifies pain. If Donna's PTSD were treated, her pain and need for medication would decrease. Failure to treat her underlying PTSD could enable a process whereby her psychological factors would be medicated with opioids (opioids are not approved to treat PTSD or other psychopathology). And it would enable her to maintain a passive role that was not helping her get better.
- A comprehensive biopsychosocial pain treatment approach was indicated. Donna was being overmedicalized and overmedicated. She clearly needed physical therapy and a gentle rehabilitation approach that would

address her fear of movement and pain. Additional medical procedures would only distract from the primary issue: Donna needed help becoming an active participant in her pain care. At that time, her psychological factors (PTSD, panic disorder with agoraphobia, and fear of movement and pain) were preventing her from engaging in active rehabilitation treatment. The recommendation was for her to first obtain treatment from a PTSD specialist, then evidence-based physical and psychological treatment for pain, before following up in 6 months.

Donna received two treatments for PTSD: prolonged exposure and eye movement desensitization and reprocessing therapy. Although she was not symptom free, she was markedly improved. She could sleep at night, was no longer hypervigilant, and was not having flashbacks. She was less reactive to pain and stress in general, and she could now tolerate relaxation without being overwhelmed and "flooded" with anxiety. She was hopeful and felt ready for the next phase of treatments that were recommended: physical therapy and cognitive behavioral therapy (CBT) for pain. She began to wonder whether she might be able to avoid the morphine pump altogether if she continued gaining positive results. She heard that some people could manage their chronic pain without opioids, and she was determined to see whether she could be one of them.

INTERVENTIONS FOR CHRONIC PAIN

Interventions for pain are varied and span a wide gamut of medical, physical, psychosocial, and complementary and alternative treatments. Each year, the American Chronic Pain Association publishes an updated consumer guide entitled *ACPA Resource Guide to Chronic Pain Management: An Integrated Guide to Medical, Interventional, Behavioral, Pharmacologic and Rehabilitation Therapies.* This consumer resource may be useful for patients and psychologists alike. The 2018 guide is freely downloadable from https://www.theacpa.org/wp-content/uploads/2018/03/ACPA_Resource_Guide_2018-Final-v2.pdf

There are hundreds of different chronic pain conditions and hundreds of medications used to treat pain. Patients will often have tried multiple medical treatments and be currently taking multiple medications to treat their pain and related symptoms. Importantly, many individuals with chronic pain have more than one pain condition, thereby adding complexity. So-called *overlapping pain conditions* are understudied despite being common (Maixner, Fillingim, Williams, Smith, & Slade, 2016).

Basic medical decision making regarding pain treatment depends on the type of pain. Pain may be classified according to the condition or the location of the pain. Table 2.1 provides examples of pain types, but neat categorizations are not always possible because of the varied etiologies of pain. For instance, back pain is the most common type of chronic pain; this label references the bodily location of the pain, though chronic back pain may be classified as joint pain (e.g., due to problems in the facets), of neuropathic origin (e.g., postsurgical chronic pain), of musculoskeletal origin (e.g., myofascial pain), or a combination of multiple factors and contributors.

Table 2.1

Pain Types and Examples

Pain types	Examples and definition
Neuropathic	Facial nerve problems (e.g., trigeminal neuralgia); pain caused from chemotherapy, HIV, shingles, spine surgery
Malignant	Cancer pain
Nonmalignant	Any pain not related to cancer
Visceral	Irritable bowel disease, gut pain
Central	Poststroke pain, multiple sclerosis
Joint	Osteoarthritis, rheumatoid arthritis
Myofascial or muscular	Fibromyalgia
Iatrogenic	Caused from medical intervention
Idiopathic	Of unknown origin

Medical Treatments for Pain

Standard medical treatment for pain typically involves an evaluation by a primary care physician. Even if a person with pain first seeks medical attention at a hospital emergency department, they will later find their way to their primary care physician. A physician typically obtains a history and performs a physical examination. In some cases, imaging, such as X-ray, ultrasound, computed tomography scan, or magnetic resonance imaging may be ordered. These imaging tests may confirm a diagnosis or rule out a suspected diagnosis. It is tempting to place a lot of faith in a medical image. Even insurance companies are more likely to approve various medical procedures if a medical image provides evidence of need. As previously discussed, medical imaging results may correlate poorly with reports of pain. Unfortunately, patients may experience judgment or stigma by health care providers or insurance carriers, and patients may be told (or encode) that their pain "is all in their head." Such pejorative statements can leave patients feeling blamed, shamed, and disenfranchised from their health care providers or the medical system. Malingering may be present in a sizable minority of patients who are seeking compensation for pain in the medico-legal context. A specialized psychological evaluation assesses for secondary gain in these cases. The most helpful approach is to assume that all pain is real, regardless of the evidence, diagnosis, or etiology of one's pain condition. Behavioral health professionals play an important role in validating the patient experience of pain and helping them understand their pain is not their fault.

Oral Medications

There are more than 200 different types of medications used to treat pain. Table 2.2 presents a brief list of the most common types of medication classes and medications used for chronic pain. With the exception of some of the nonsteroidal anti-inflammatory drugs, all the pain medications listed require a physician's prescription.

Antidepressants as Pain Treatment. Serotonin and norepinephrine reuptake inhibitors (SNRIs) are a specific class of antidepressant medications that are commonly prescribed to treat neuropathic pain (Attal

Table 2.2

Pain Medication Types and Examples

	Examples	
Medication type	Generic names	Brand names
Selective serotonin norepinephrine reuptake inhibitors	duloxetine venlafaxine	Cymbalta Effexor
Nerve pain anticonvulsant	gabapentin pregabalin	Neurontin Lyrica
Nonsteroidal anti-inflammatory drugs	celecoxib diclofenac ibuprofen naproxen aspirin	Celebrex Cambia, Voltaren Motrin, Advil Aleve, Naprosyn
Opioids[a]	hydrocodone	Norco Vicodin Hysingla (ER)
	oxycodone	Oxycontin Percocet Roxycodone
	hydromorphone fentanyl	Dilaudid Duragesic (ER)
Muscle relaxant	baclofen	
Cannabinoids		Sativex Marinol

Note. ER = extended release.
[a]Opioids are controlled substances.

et al., 2010). Patients may sometimes express concern about being prescribed an antidepressant for pain because they may misinterpret the prescription as meaning that their doctor thinks their pain is psychological. In fact, SNRIs simply modulate pain through the serotonin and norepinephrine neurotransmitters (E. M. Smith et al., 2013; Sumpton & Moulin, 2001). If patients are prescribed an SNRI for neuropathic pain, it does not mean they are depressed. However, if a patient has comorbid neuropathic pain and depression, an SNRI may dually treat both conditions.

Opioid Medications. Opioids are covered in detail in Chapter 9. However, in this chapter on pain medications, it is important to note that pain is rarely eliminated with medication, and for this reason, the term *painkiller* is a misnomer. Attempts to reach a "pain-free" state through medications such as opioids can promote medication overuse, risky doses, side effects, and addiction. Overuse of medications invites a host of other problems that can worsen pain and promote increasing medical complexity and *polypharmacy* (multiple medications being coprescribed, often to treat the side effects of the previously prescribed medication). Figure 2.1 illustrates how opioids may lead to greater medical complexity when new prescriptions are written to treat opioid side effects. Increasing prescriptions and an overfocus on medications perpetuates a false belief that there is a little one can do to reduce one's pain and suffering. A key message is that medication can be one part of a comprehensive pain care plan that seeks to reduce the impact of chronic pain by helping people self-manage their pain, reduce their suffering, and live richer lives even if a degree of pain remains. Chapter 9 provides detail on opioids, medical, and psychological factors.

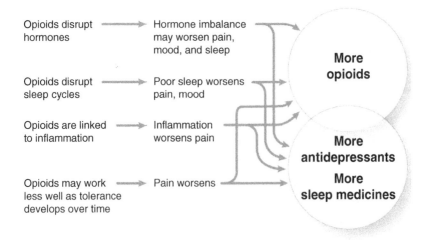

Figure 2.1

How opioids can lead to more pain and more medications. From *Less Pain, Fewer Pills: Avoid the Dangers of Prescription Opioids and Gain Control Over Chronic Pain*, by B. Darnall, 2014, p. 17. Copyright 2014 by Bull Publishing Company. Reprinted with permission.

Common Medical Procedures for Pain

Some commonly used medical procedures for pain include

- injections (used for diagnostic and therapeutic purposes)
  - trigger point injections
  - epidural steroid injections
  - nerve blocks (local anesthetic)
  - sympathetic blocks
- implanted devices
  - spinal cord stimulators
  - intrathecal medication pumps
- intravenous medication infusions (lidocaine, ketamine)
- Denervation (e.g., radiofrequency, cryo, chemical)

Common Topical Medications

Some commonly used topical medications for pain (skin delivery, prescription) include

- lidocaine patch
- fentanyl (opioid patch)
- Butrans patch (Suboxone patch)

Over-the-Counter Oral Medications and Supplements

Some commonly used over-the-counter oral medications and supplements include

- nonsteroidal anti-inflammatory medications
- acetaminophen
- aspirin
- herbal supplements (e.g., curcumin, turmeric, ginger)

Nonmedical Treatments for Pain

Common Nonmedical Pain Treatments

The following are some commonly used nonmedical pain treatments:

- physical therapy and rehabilitation
- movement and exercise

- acupuncture
- transcutaneous electrical nerve stimulation
- massage
- occupational therapy
- chiropractic
- gentle yoga
- Reiki

Common Psychobehavioral Treatments for Chronic Pain

The following are some common psychobehavioral treatments for pain:

- CBT
- mindfulness-based stress reduction
- mindfulness meditation
- acceptance and commitment therapy ("contextual CBT")
- chronic pain self-management
- relaxation response
- pain education
- biofeedback
- hypnosis

Novel Treatments

The following are some novel approaches used in the treatment of pain:

- transmagnetic cranial stimulation
- virtual reality

Physical Treatment for Chronic Pain

Appropriate movement is integral to pain management and functional rehabilitation. What constitutes appropriate movement is dependent on each individual's medical, physical, and psychosocial characteristics. Evaluation with a physical therapist who has expertise in treating chronic pain is ideal. Importantly, like psychologists and even physicians, many physical therapists—including those with advanced degrees—may not be well trained in chronic pain treatment principles. Good chronic pain physical therapists are knowledgeable about basic psychological factors that can impede engagement in movement and self-management, such as fear of pain and fear-avoidance behaviors. Physical therapists can use various skills (Diener, Kargela, & Louw, 2016) such as providing relevant pain education and relaxation coaching to help clients through their fear as they engage in gentle movements (George, 2006; George, Fritz, Bialosky, & Donald, 2003). Such combined approaches can help extinguish some of the psychobehavioral barriers that may be contributing to disability and further pain. Figure 2.2, in a graphical representation of the fear-avoidance model, reproduced from Vlaeyen and Linton (2000), depicts the critical interplay between psychological factors and movement in pain cycles and disability. Fear-based psychobehavioral factors lead to activity avoidance, disuse, and disability, and a bidirectional relationship is established. Recovery occurs by confronting one's fear of movement. Although

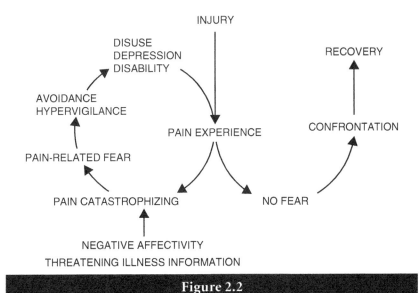

Figure 2.2

The fear-avoidance cycle. From "Fear-Avoidance and Its Consequences in Chronic Musculoskeletal Pain: A State of the Art," by J. W. Vlaeyen and S. J. Linton, 2000, *Pain*, 85, p. 329. Copyright 2000 by the International Association for the Study of Pain. Reprinted with permission.

no small feat, a skilled team that includes a psychologist and physical therapist can provide patients with the roadmap and support to begin moving forward with functional goals.

DOUGLAS'S BACK PAIN PROBLEM

Douglas is a 45-year-old man who was working as a manager at the largest hardware supply retailer in the United States. Several years ago, he injured his back while helping a colleague lift some stock onto the store shelves. What seemed to be a simple injury has not been simple at all. For Douglas, the injury has been life changing. In the past 3 years he has had two operations on his back. He was prescribed opioids for his postsurgical pain, and then they were continued indefinitely. Douglas is dismayed that the surgeries have not helped as much as everyone expected. He had a brief course of physical therapy to help him recover after the surgery and get back to work. He went a few times but found traveling to his appointments was difficult. Plus, the sessions were painful, and he was worried about reinjuring his back. He also did not connect well with his therapist, so he stopped going and just continued with the pills while waiting for his full recovery. The opioid medication was just taking the edge off his pain, but the tradeoffs were severe constipation and erectile dysfunction side effects. Even with opioids the pain was definitely still there, and it was preventing him from doing much at all. He was reassigned to an administrative desk job at work. Although he was grateful to still be working, he was becoming increasingly concerned because he was now finding that sitting was making his pain worse. Before standing and lifting hurt, but now that sitting hurt too, the only thing left was lying down! Before his injury, Douglas was an athletic and fit 45-year-old. Now he felt like a fragile old man with health problems. He did not feel like socializing or dating because he felt embarrassed about his medical condition and how little he could do.

Douglas's doctor was unhappy with his recovery and persistent pain after surgery. It was clear he needed a higher level of care and coordinated support. She referred him to a multidisciplinary pain clinic where he began treatment with a physical therapist and a pain psychologist. His care plan was coordinated to address several important therapeutic targets. First, he needed to understand which movements and exercises would help him recover and gain strength and function. He needed to understand what level of discomfort was expected and safe for him. He needed help in learning to interpret his body's signals and to trust his body and his therapists. In working with his physical therapist and psychologist, he learned that just because he felt pain did not mean he was injuring his back. He learned how to begin moving again. He learned that moving was the key to his recovery and to managing pain, and this information alone helped him feel better emotionally too. He felt relieved that he had a treatment team to help him get where he wanted to be. His psychologist helped him with setting realistic goals, and he learned about daily self-management practices that would help with positive mood and pain management. Once he gained traction with physical therapy and psychological treatment, Douglas and his doctor began discussing a plan to wean him slowly from the opioids. Because his pain was neuropathic, his pain doctor recommended he begin an SNRI, such as Cymbalta or Effexor. It was hoped that by stopping the opioids Douglas's constipation and erectile dysfunction would resolve and that the SNRI might have the happy side effect of bolstering his mood further.

KEY POINTS

- Having a general understanding of medical pain treatments is valuable for understanding the patient experience, the range of treatments used, and factors that may affect medical and psychotherapeutic treatment decision making.
- Pain diagnoses, comorbidities, and psychological, historical, and other individual factors influence a patient's candidacy for various medical pain treatments.
- Examples of various medical pain treatments include medications, surgery, spinal cord stimulator or other form of neuromodulation, injections, and nerve procedures.
- Physical therapy and rehabilitation approaches are important components of pain treatment.

RESOURCES

This free consumer resource may be useful for patients and psychologists alike:

American Chronic Pain Association. (2018). *ACPA resource guide to chronic pain management: An integrated guide to medical, interventional, behavioral, pharmacologic and rehabilitation therapies.* Retrieved from https://www.theacpa.org/wp-content/uploads/2018/03/ACPA_Resource_Guide_2018-Final-v2.pdf

Free publication:

Kopf, A., & Patel, N. B. (Eds.). (2010). *Guide to pain management in low-resource settings.* Seattle, WA: International Association for the Treatment of Pain. Retrieved from https://s3.amazonaws.com/rdcms-iasp/files/production/public/Content/ContentFolders/Publications2/FreeBooks/Guide_to_Pain_Management_in_Low-Resource_Settings.pdf

Integrative pain management:

Stein, T. (2016). *The everything guide to integrative pain management: Conventional and alternative therapies for managing pain.* Avon, MA: Adams Media.

3

Depression, Anxiety, and Posttraumatic Stress Disorder

D epression and anxiety disorders are the most common mental health conditions that co-occur with chronic pain. Individuals with chronic pain are more likely to acquire a mood or anxiety disorder as a consequence of the pain and related life changes, such as sleep disorders, disability, and social isolation (Harris, 2014). On the flip side, having a mental health condition or behavioral health challenges (e.g., insomnia, poor sleep) increases the likelihood of developing future chronic pain (Bair, Robinson, Katon, & Kroenke, 2003; Carroll, Cassidy, & Côté, 2004; Generaal, Vogelzangs, Penninx, & Dekker, 2017; Kessler, Chiu, Demler, & Walters, 2005). Indeed, psychological conditions and chronic pain are often bidirectionally related, with literature suggesting a model of mutual maintenance (Asmundson & Katz, 2009). Psychological treatment for chronic pain necessarily involves assessing patients for current mental health conditions that contribute to greater pain and suffering from it.

http://dx.doi.org/10.1037/0000104-004
Psychological Treatment for Patients With Chronic Pain, by B. D. Darnall

DEPRESSION

It is estimated that 40% to 60% of individuals with chronic pain have co-occurring depression, with the high prevalence of comorbidity prompting the coining of the term *depression–pain dyad* (Bair et al., 2003). Patients may have a primary mood disorder, or the mood disorder may arise as a consequence of chronic pain and may be coded as a mood disorder due to a general medical condition. Common correlates of chronic pain, sleep disturbance and feelings of helplessness, are also depressive symptoms that contribute to a diagnosis of major depression. Finally, even patients who do not meet formal criteria for major depression are likely to have some depressive symptoms related to their pain. Independent of a clinical diagnosis, frustration about pain-related interference and functional limitations are common experiences and important therapeutic targets to improve emotional experience and to prevent deterioration of mood.

Depression predicts a greater likelihood to acquire chronic pain, and once chronic pain is established, concurrent depression is associated with greater pain intensity, disability, and poorer outcomes for pain (Roh et al., 2012). Pain and depression independently contribute to decreased physical and social activities, and their combination may greatly compound disability and poor outcomes compared with either one in isolation (Ohayon, 2004). Depression may be particularly vexing in the context of pain because it can impede a patient's engagement in crucial pain rehabilitation activities, thereby maintaining and worsening disability, pain, and depression. Finally, moderate symptoms of depression have been associated with a greater risk of pain medication misuse, even in the absence of a history of substance use disorder (Grattan, Sullivan, Saunders, Campbell, & Von Korff, 2012). The striking prevalence and negative impacts of depression and depressive symptoms in chronic pain underscore the need for proper assessment and treatment.

Treatment

Effective psychological and behavioral treatments for pain may be dually beneficial for improving mood. For instance, appropriate activation, movement, and exercise are excellent behavioral medicine for pain and depression (Rainville et al., 2004). Moreover, general self-care practices also serve to improve pain and mood alike. Mental health professionals can guide clients to develop appropriate and achievable activity and self-care goals. When possible, weekly therapy sessions are recommended to support patients in their greater engagement in pain self-management activities.

Depressive rumination may predispose patients to ruminate on their pain. Pain rumination is one component of a broader pattern of pain catastrophizing, discussed in detail in Chapter 4. Pain rumination is an important therapeutic target because it serves to entrain neural patterns (brain function) on pain and related emotional distress—both serving to amplify pain processing in the nervous system. Amplification and suffering can promote feelings of helplessness, and helplessness is shared criteria for depression and pain catastrophizing. Effective treatment for depression and pain must address pain catastrophizing because it is common to both.

Cognitive behavioral therapy for pain (pain-CBT) is an evidence-based psychological treatment that is primarily effective for reducing pain catastrophizing and disability. Although individual studies have shown pain-CBT improves mood, a meta-analysis of 35 different studies found that pain-CBT is beneficial for depression only when compared with usual care (effects were lost when compared with an active control; Williams, Eccleston, & Morley, 2012). However, a recent study of almost 400 veterans revealed that pain-CBT was effective for reducing pain, catastrophizing, depression, and disability.

A variant of pain-CBT, acceptance and commitment therapy (ACT), has been shown to reduce depression and anxiety and improve self-efficacy and activity engagement (Hughes, Clark, Colclough, Dale, & McMillan, 2017) and function (Vowles, Witkiewitz, Levell, Sowden, & Ashworth, 2017). It is important to note that in chronic pain research, ACT is typically delivered in the context of multidisciplinary pain treatment programs, and the goals of treatment are specific to managing pain.

Medication Considerations

As noted in Chapter 2, serotonin and norepinephrine reuptake inhibitors (SNRIs) are antidepressant medications that are effective for neuropathic pain. In patients with neuropathic pain and comorbid depression, SNRI treatment may be beneficial for both. For patients currently taking other classes of antidepressant medication, such as selective serotonin reuptake inhibitors, prescribers may slowly taper and switch them to an SNRI. Psychological treatment remains highly relevant to those prescribed antidepressants. The general depression literature has suggested that combining psychological and antidepressant treatment can yield greater effects than either one alone (Cuijpers, 2014; de Jonghe et al., 2004; de Jonghe, Kool, van Aalst, Dekker, & Peen, 2001; Karyotaki et al., 2016).

Although Chapter 9 covers opioids in greater detail, a few considerations specific to depression bear mentioning here. Individuals with chronic pain and depression are more likely to be prescribed opioids at higher doses and take them longer than individuals with chronic pain who are not depressed. Several unintended consequences of opioids may serve to worsen mood. For instance, opioids alter hormones and erode sleep quality, two factors that may facilitate depression and pain. Some research has shown that long-term opioid use predicts new onset of major depression (Salas et al., 2017; Scherrer et al., 2017). For these reasons, it can be useful to assess the timing of opioid initiation or dose increases and mood symptoms.

Other clinical considerations involve medication-taking behavior. Depressed individuals are at greater risk of misusing opioids or using opioids at higher doses (Edlund, Martin, Fan, Braden, et al., 2010; Edlund, Martin, Fan, Devries, et al., 2010; Edlund, Steffick, Hudson, Harris, & Sullivan, 2007; Grattan et al., 2012; M. D. Sullivan et al., 2010). Risks may compound when additional psychological factors and comorbidities are present, such as history of trauma, posttraumatic stress disorder (PTSD), and smoking (Hooten, Shi, Gazelka, & Warner, 2011; K. Z. Smith, Smith, Cercone, McKee, & Homish, 2016).

Assessment of Depression and Pain: Special Considerations

- Assessment for depression in chronic pain is accomplished with general methods and screening tools (e.g., clinical interview, Beck Depression Inventory–II, Patient Health Questionnaire–9, Center for Epidemiological

Studies Depression Scale). When assessing for depressive symptoms, note that some depression screening tools, such as the Beck Depression Inventory, have a greater number of somatic items and therefore may yield higher—yet still valid—scores in individuals with medical conditions and chronic pain (Knaster, Estlander, Karlsson, Kaprio, & Kalso, 2016).

- Assess for relevant depression qualifiers. Adjustment disorder with depression may be an appropriate diagnosis.
- In cases where suicidality is present, assess for current or stockpiled pain medications and other prescriptions that are potential means of self-harm.

ANXIETY DISORDERS

Chronic pain and anxiety disorders (generalized anxiety disorder, obsessive-compulsive disorder, pain disorder with agoraphobia, and PTSD) commonly co-occur. The estimated 12-month prevalence of anxiety disorder or severe anxiety exceeds 50% for patients with chronic pain conditions such as fibromyalgia, abdominal pain, and temporomandibular joint disorder (Arnold et al., 2006; Burris, Cyders, de Leeuw, Smith, & Carlson, 2009). Evidence supports bidirectional etiologies for anxiety and chronic pain. For instance, individuals with migraine have a two- to three-fold likelihood of having a diagnosed anxiety disorder compared with healthy individuals (Saunders, Merikangas, Low, Von Korff, & Kessler, 2008). Chronic pain appears to confer risk of developing a de novo anxiety disorder. Researchers who conducted a prospective population study found that among individuals with chronic pain and no history of anxiety disorder, 15% to 16% went on to develop an anxiety disorder during the 2-year follow-up period (Gerrits, van Oppen, van Marwijk, Penninx, & van der Horst, 2014). A greater number of painful body sites was found to associate directly with the development of anxiety and to predict a more complicated course (Gerrits et al., 2012). Other researchers have shown that experiencing pain after a motor vehicle collision predicts the later development of PTSD (Khodadadi-Hassankiadeh, Dehghan Nayeri, Shahsavari, Yousefzadeh-Chabok, & Haghani, 2017).

Viewed from the other direction, anxiety appears to confer risk of the development of chronic pain. For instance, research has suggested that individuals with an anxiety disorder are twice as likely to develop migraine headache relative to individuals without anxiety (Bruffaerts et al., 2015). Anxiety is also a risk factor for the development and persistence of back pain (Picavet, Vlaeyen, & Schouten, 2002), pain following surgery (Theunissen, Peters, Bruce, Gramke, & Marcus, 2012), and pain following physical and psychological trauma (McLean, Clauw, Abelson, & Liberzon, 2005). It is hypothesized that anxiety may facilitate the progression of pain by contributing to maladaptive cognitive, emotional, and behavioral responses to the early stages of pain that are known to impede recovery.

Angela's Story

Angela is a 45-year-old woman with chronic left shoulder pain that began when she sustained an injury in a car accident 3 years prior.[1] She worked as a grocery clerk at the time and was rear-ended by a fast-moving car while driving to her store one morning. She was diagnosed with whiplash and a shoulder injury from being caught in the seatbelt. Angela had a history of panic attacks that stretched back to college; the worst of it was in her late 20s when she was going through a bad breakup. She had some social anxiety as well but nothing that affected her functioning, outside of avoiding large parties and gatherings. After her car accident, her anxiety flared up. She was not having nightmares or flashbacks, but she did not feel safe in a car anymore. Her neck and shoulder were hurting, and she found herself constantly focusing on her pain. Her doctor assured her that normal healing was taking place, but she worried that something else must be really wrong—it just hurt too much. She found herself constantly monitoring for pain and trying to evaluate whether it was getting worse. Early on, she was given shoulder exercises to do at home, but they made her pain worse. She was struggling with anxiety about doing the exercises, and finally, she just stopped doing them altogether. Her doctor declared

---

[1]The case example used in this chapter is fictitious or has been disguised to protect confidentiality.

that her neck injury and shoulder tear had healed, but then why did she still have so much pain? Three years later she still could not use her arm as she used to, and her short-term work disability turned into long-term disability. She was spending her days at home mostly trying to stay comfortable and avoiding anything that would cause her even more pain. As a result, she was barely using her left arm at all.

Angela's case illustrates several useful points. First, she had anxiety before her accident, so she was primed to have her anxiety flare up after her accident. Anxiety, greater somatic awareness, and hypervigilance all magnify the experience of pain, with increased attention to pain, exaggerated pain responses, and activity avoidance behaviors that impede rehabilitation and recovery. Although Angela's avoidance (stopping her rehab exercises) helped her gain some short-term relief from pain and anxiety, it contributed to greater pain and anxiety over time. Anxiety and avoidance of anxiety-provoking stimuli often go hand in hand. In Angela's case, anxiety about her pain led her to avoid the very activities that would have helped her recover. Mental health professionals play a critical role in treating underlying anxiety—and addressing anxiety about pain—so that patients can use skills to calm their nervous system and be better able to move forward with appropriate treatments. After her accident, Angela would have benefited from working with a psychologist skilled in treating anxiety and a physical therapist who was skilled in addressing fear-avoidance behaviors. Important components of clinical care include assessing and addressing any psychobehavioral barriers—such as anxiety—that may impede patients' engagement in pain rehabilitation, pain self-management, and good self-care practices.

Assessment for Anxiety in Chronic Pain: Special Considerations

- Assess patients for comorbid pain and anxiety. If you are comfortable treating anxiety, choose anxiety as your therapeutic target. Explore how anxiety may be affecting the experience of pain, fear of pain, and avoidance behaviors.
- Individuals who are medically cleared for activity may still avoid the activity out of fear that their pain will worsen. Slow, graded exposure

to the activity may help patients increase their confidence and function, while simultaneously extinguishing fear. Slow increases in activity levels are key in preventing pain flares. A physical therapist skilled in treating chronic pain can help engage patients in appropriate movement therapies and in vivo graded exposure to address their fears in the treatment session (Woods & Asmundson, 2008).

■ Anxiety about pain may also counterproductively motivate patients to push beyond their physical limits and engage in poor pacing, thereby contributing to their cycle of pain (see Figure 3.1).

Patients may find themselves caught in a tumultuous pattern that includes wild fluctuations of over- and underactivity and anxiety serving to maintain both. Helping patients establish realistic goals and levels of activity that are appropriate for their current body (not their prepain body) is essential for managing pain, reducing distress, and helping them learn to deliver best self-care. For this reason, pain-specific psychological treatments, such as pain-CBT, ACT, and chronic pain self-management, all encourage appropriate goal setting for activities that reflect the person's

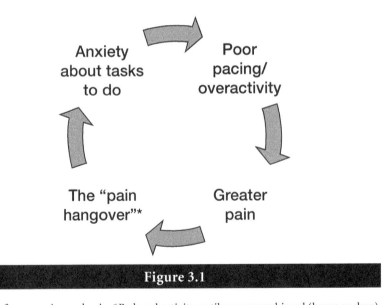

Figure 3.1

Cycle of poor pacing and pain. *Reduced activity until recovery achieved (hours or days).

current status and good activity-pacing principles to ensure an activity balance that extinguishes the negative pain cycles.

POSTTRAUMATIC STRESS DISORDER

Though PTSD falls under the broad umbrella of anxiety disorders, it is given separate consideration here because of the unique effect of psychological and physical trauma on the experience of pain. Like depression and other anxiety disorders, co-occurrence of chronic pain and PTSD negatively affects the course of both disorders. For instance, individuals with comorbid PTSD and chronic pain report greater pain, disability, and affective distress. Compared with individuals who do not fulfill criteria for PTSD or have no history of trauma, individuals with PTSD report significantly higher levels of pain interference, kinesiophobia (fear of movement), anxiety, and depression and significantly lower levels of life control (Åkerblom, Perrin, Rivano Fischer, & McCracken, 2017).

Up to 75% of individuals seeking treatment for PTSD report having chronic pain. Viewed from the other angle, among patients seeking treatment for chronic pain, more than 70% report having been exposed to at least one traumatic event, and roughly 30% have been diagnosed with comorbid PTSD (Åkerblom et al., 2017), compared with 3.5% in the general population (Kessler et al., 2005). In other words, individuals with chronic pain are 8.5 times as likely to have PTSD than the general population. Chronic pain may be an antecedent to the development of PTSD symptoms, even if the etiology is nontraumatic. The bidirectional relationship between pain and PTSD suggests shared neurobiology (Scioli-Salter et al., 2015). Pain—a hardwired signal of physical threat—can serve to trigger and worsen PTSD symptoms such as reexperiencing the trauma, and conversely PTSD-related hypervigilance and muscle tension can serve to maintain and worsen pain.

The traumatic incident that led to the development of PTSD may have involved physical harm and pain, thereby further entwining the two disorders into a negative psychosensory experience that is self-reinforcing and highly distressing. New onset pain may trigger latent trauma, possibly even from childhood, to surface during a particularly vulnerable time. Finally, some research has suggested that even without PTSD, trauma exposure is sufficient to increase pain sensitivity—an index of lasting changes in the nervous system—and may partially explain the association between trauma and chronic pain (Tesarz et al., 2015).

Treatment

PTSD is a known precursor to substance use disorder, with some research showing that trauma cues (e.g., pain) are associated with greater cravings (Simpson, Stappenbeck, Varra, Moore, & Kaysen, 2012). Individuals with pain and PTSD should be assessed and monitored for substance use; whenever possible, opioids should be avoided because of the high risk of misuse and addiction.

Because PTSD necessarily involves an exaggerated response to threat-related cues—such as pain—treatment for chronic pain must include PTSD treatment in individuals who have this diagnosis. Research has suggested that greater PTSD severity directly relates to pain sensitivity and poor ability to use adaptive cognitive skills to reduce one's experience of pain (i.e., poor self-modulation of pain; Defrin, Lahav, & Solomon, 2017). Learning to reduce attention and reactivity to pain are critical components of psychological treatment for pain. However, hallmarks of PTSD—hyperarousal and hypervigilance for threat—can foster catastrophizing and fear of pain, thereby impeding one's ability to learn and successfully apply basic pain psychology skills. Patients fearful of addressing their trauma and PTSD symptoms may be more willing to focus on pain or depressive symptoms; however, traction with pain management is likely to be limited if PTSD symptoms are not treated.

Interesting findings from research in veterans with pain and PTSD have suggested that activity and exercise—in spite of severe chronic pain—may temper PTSD symptoms (Bourn, Sexton, Porter, & Rauch, 2016). As long as good pacing principles are applied, activity and exercise are likely to also reduce pain, sleep problems, and underlying depressive symptoms. An important aspect of psychological treatment for chronic pain involves helping patients effect the relaxation response to gain control over how pain affects brain and body (see Chapter 5). Individuals with severe PTSD may not tolerate relaxation because it may trigger a flooding of anxiety and potentially a panic attack. Effective treatment for PTSD and symptom reduction may allow patients to use relaxation as a pain management skill, calm nervous system activity, and reduce the impact of pain.

Assessment and Treatment: Special Considerations

- Routinely screen patients with either PTSD or chronic pain for the presence of the other condition. Assessment for co-occurrence may reveal an important latent therapeutic target.
- Pain is associated with the development of PTSD symptoms, even in the absence of other trauma.
- Eye movement desensitization reprocessing (EMDR) therapy is an evidence-based treatment for PTSD that has also shown promise as a treatment for chronic pain; however, additional studies are needed before definitive treatment recommendations can be made for EMDR as a treatment for stand-alone chronic pain (Tesarz et al., 2014). However, given its efficacy for treating PTSD, EMDR may yield dual benefits for patients with comorbid chronic pain.
- Individuals with PTSD and chronic pain are at greatly increased risk of substance use disorder. Assess for substance use, as well as use of pain medications to determine whether self-medication of psychological distress is occurring through the use of alcohol, marijuana, illicit substances, or prescription medications.
- If the use of relaxation skills at home causes increased anxiety (e.g., flooding and/or panic attacks), the patient requires a higher level of care including individual psychotherapy with a PTSD specialist.

KEY POINTS

- Psychological disorders commonly co-occur with pain and have a significant impact on the trajectory of pain and response to pain treatment.

- Anxiety and depression prevalence estimates for individuals with chronic pain are 50% each, suggesting substantial psychological comorbidity with pain.
- Depression and anxiety disorders may precede pain or can develop as a consequence of living with ongoing pain.
- Behavioral factors, such as poor pacing or fear avoidance, can contribute to pain cycles and pain progression. Addressing underlying psychological factors can facilitate adaptive behavior change.
- Key psychological symptoms, such as rumination on pain, hypervigilance for pain, feelings of helplessness, and sleep disturbance, are important therapeutic targets that can dually improve physical and pain status through changes in behavior (e.g., reducing fear avoidance), attention, and self-regulation.
- Up to 75% of individuals seeking treatment for PTSD report having chronic pain.
- Screening and treatment for depression, anxiety, and PTSD is important in patients with chronic pain. Likewise, assessing for pain is essential in all patients and in particular those with psychological distress or disorders.

RESOURCES

PTSD clinical checklist:

U.S. Department of Veterans Affairs. (2017). *PTSD checklist for* DSM–5 *(PCL-5)*. Retrieved from https://www.ptsd.va.gov/professional/assessment/adult-sr/ptsd-checklist.asp

Measure and scoring: PTSD CheckList—Civilian Version (PCL-C). Available at https://www.mirecc.va.gov/docs/visn6/3_PTSD_CheckList_and_Scoring.pdf

Free mental health therapist guide on chronic pain and PTSD:

DeCarvalho, L. T. (2016). *The experience of chronic pain and PTSD: A guide for health care providers*. Retrieved from https://www.ptsd.va.gov/professional/co-occurring/chronic-pain-ptsd-providers.asp

Neurobiology of pain and PTSD (review):

Scioli-Salter, E. R., Forman, D. E., Otis, J. D., Gregor, K., Valovski, I., & Rasmusson, A. M. (2015). The shared neuroanatomy and neurobiology of comorbid chronic pain and PTSD: Therapeutic implications. *The Clinical Journal of Pain, 31,* 363–374. http://dx.doi.org/10.1097/AJP.0000000000000115

PTSD and substance use disorder (free PubMed Central article):

Berenz, E. C., & Coffey, S. F. (2012). Treatment of co-occurring posttraumatic stress disorder and substance use disorders. *Current Psychiatry Reports, 14,* 469–477. http://dx.doi.org/10.1007/s11920-012-0300-0

4

Pain-Specific Psychological Factors

As discussed in Chapter 1, general psychobehavioral factors are integral to the experience of pain. Chapter 3 expanded the focus to the role of major psychological comorbidities and pain. Chapter 4 extends the conversation beyond psychological diagnoses and covers several critical pain-specific psychobehavioral factors that influence pain, treatment needs, and treatment outcomes. The most impactful pain-specific psychobehavioral factors are pain catastrophizing, fear of pain, fear of movement (*kinesiophobia*), pain-related anxiety, and pain self-efficacy.

PAIN CATASTROPHIZING

Pain catastrophizing is a pattern of negative cognitive and emotional responses to pain and includes rumination on pain, the magnification of pain, and feelings of helplessness about pain. Often there is a focus on the "worst-case scenario": "What happens if my pain gets worse?" or "What if

http://dx.doi.org/10.1037/0000104-005
Psychological Treatment for Patients With Chronic Pain, by B. D. Darnall

> Pain catastrophizing is often more important than medical variables. For instance, catastrophizing is the most powerful predictor for back pain disability 1 year after new-onset back pain.

something is seriously wrong with me?" Pain catastrophizing is most commonly measured with the Catastrophizing subscale of the Coping Skills Questionnaire (Rosenstiel & Keefe, 1983) or with the Pain Catastrophizing Scale (M. J. L. Sullivan, Bishop, & Pivik, 1995).

The Pain Catastrophizing Scale

The Pain Catastrophizing Scale (PCS; M. J. L. Sullivan et al., 1995) is presented in Figure 4.1. The 13 items are summed to arrive at a total PCS score, ranging from 0 to 52. Individuals seeking specialty care from a pain clinic tend to have mean PCS scores of about 25 or so and can benefit from treatment. Other studies have shown that PCS scores in the range of 13 to 16 are associated with poor outcomes after surgery and a greater likelihood of having an opioid prescription (Helmerhorst, Vranceanu, Vrahas, Smith, & Ring, 2014; Sharifzadeh et al., 2017). Scores of 10 or less on the PCS have no clear associations with the development of chronic pain or negative outcomes for existing chronic pain; therefore, a PCS score of 10 is a recommended therapeutic target. Note that the PCS quantifies the frequency of negative thoughts and feelings about pain. It is normal to have occasional negative thoughts when one is experiencing pain. Experiencing them often or continuously when in pain indicates a clear need for intervention.

Left untreated, pain catastrophizing exerts an array of negative impacts. For instance, greater levels of pain catastrophizing are associated with

- emotional distress,
- muscle and joint tenderness (Severeijns, Vlaeyen, van den Hout, & Weber, 2001),
- muscle tension,
- pain intensity (Sharifzadeh et al., 2017),

	Not at all	To a slight degree	To a moderate degree	To a great degree	All the time
1. I worry all the time about whether the pain will end.	0	1	2	3	4
2. I feel I can't go on.	0	1	2	3	4
3. The pain is terrible and I think it's never going to get any better.	0	1	2	3	4
4. The pain is awful and I feel that it overwhelms me.	0	1	2	3	4
5. I feel I can't stand the pain anymore.	0	1	2	3	4
6. I become afraid that the pain will get worse.	0	1	2	3	4
7. I keep thinking of other painful events.	0	1	2	3	4
8. I anxiously want the pain to go away.	0	1	2	3	4
9. I can't seem to keep thoughts of pain out of my mind.	0	1	2	3	4
10. I keep thinking about how much it hurts.	0	1	2	3	4
11. I keep thinking about how badly I want the pain to stop.	0	1	2	3	4
12. There's nothing I can do to reduce the intensity of the pain.	0	1	2	3	4
13. I wonder whether something serious may happen.	0	1	2	3	4

Figure 4.1

Pain Catastrophizing Scale. Instructions (adapted for chronic pain): Consider the types of thoughts and feelings that you have when you experience pain. Listed are 13 statements describing different thoughts and feelings that may be associated with pain. Using the scale, indicate the degree to which you have these thoughts and feelings when you are experiencing pain. Reprinted from "The Pain Catastrophizing Scale: Development and Validation," by M. J. L. Sullivan, S. R. Bishop, and J. Pivik, 1995, *Psychological Assessment*, 7, p. 526. Copyright 1995 by the American Psychological Association.

- pain-related disability (Abbott, Tyni-Lenné, & Hedlund, 2011; Casey, Feyer, & Cameron, 2011; Severeijns et al., 2001),
- poorer response to medical treatment for pain (Burns, Glenn, Bruehl, Harden, & Lofland, 2003; Wertli et al., 2014), and
- postsurgical pain intensity and opioid use (Helmerhorst et al., 2014) and delayed recovery from surgery (Vranceanu, Jupiter, Mudgal, & Ring, 2010).

Pain rumination is one component of pain catastrophizing (e.g., "I can't seem to keep it out of my mind," "I keep thinking about how badly I want the pain to stop") that indicates that an individual has their attention persistently focused on pain. Several studies have suggested that the ruminative component of pain catastrophizing is a primary driver of negative associations and outcomes (Jiang et al., 2016). Increased attention to pain is associated with greater pain and distress (Severeijns et al., 2001). It is vitally important for patients to acquire skills that can help them stop catastrophizing in the moment, shift their attention, and ultimately break their pattern of catastrophizing.

Impact of Catastrophizing on the Brain and Pain

Real-time brain scans show the difference in how the brain functions in people who are catastrophizing pain compared with those who are experiencing pain but are not catastrophizing it. To test these differences, researchers have conducted pain-testing experiments while individuals are in a brain scanner. Immediately after the pain experiment participants rate their level of catastrophizing during the pain test, and researchers correlate their catastrophizing scores with the results from their brain scans. People who score higher on real-time pain catastrophizing have different brain patterns than those who do not: Their scans show that regions of the brain associated with pain processing light up. Specifically, the brain regions that light up are associated with greater attention to pain and pain-related distress. These studies reveal that persistent attention to pain—and focusing on how awful it is—amplifies pain in the nervous system (Seminowicz & Davis, 2006). Individuals cannot change their medically diagnosed chronic pain condition, but they can learn critical skills that allow them to calm their nervous systems and direct their attention away from pain. In doing so, pain processing is dampened, and suffering from pain is lessened.

Pain Catastrophizing Changes the Brain

Importantly, pain catastrophizing alters the way the brain functions such that even when individuals are at rest and not in pain, their brains are primed for future pain (Hubbard et al., 2014; Jiang et al., 2016). It is thought that a persistent pattern of catastrophizing entrains the brain to have heightened awareness and negative responses so that stimuli are more likely to be felt as painful or more painful. This phenomenon is similar to a standard confirmatory bias, wherein people who expect something negative are more likely to experience it because they are looking for it, but in this case the brain is hard-wired to find pain because the neural patterns are well trained and automatic. Research shows that catastrophizing is also strongly associated with changes in the structure of the brain, such that people who catastrophize show atrophy in the regions of the brain associated with pain control (pain modulation), including the dorsolateral prefrontal cortex (Seminowicz et al., 2013). The science on catastrophizing is strong: Catastrophizing increases pain and changes neural function and is associated with lasting brain changes that lead to greater future pain (Hubbard et al., 2014; Jiang et al., 2016). In a testament to the basic principles of neuroplasticity, just as the brain can be trained toward amplified pain, the brain can also be trained in the other direction—away

Pain catastrophizing alters the structure of the brain. Pain catastrophizing also alters the way the brain functions when one is not in pain or catastrophizing. Alterations in the resting-state brain networks suggest that catastrophizing primes responsivity and attention to future pain.

from pain. Prospective cognitive behavioral therapy for pain (pain-CBT) research has shown that posttreatment reductions in pain catastrophizing are associated with significant adaptive structural brain changes—gray matter volumetric increases in the regions of the brain associated with pain control (including prefrontal and posterior parietal cortices)—that correlate with patient reports of improved pain control (Seminowicz et al., 2013). Seminowicz et al. (2013) posited that the observed posttreatment gray matter volumetric increases reflect greater top-down control over pain and cognitive reappraisal of pain and that changes in somatosensory cortices reflect alterations in the perception of noxious signals—a hypothesis that directly dovetails with the cognitive skills patients acquire in pain-CBT (see Chapter 6).

Although distraction can be a useful technique to help break catastrophizing thought cycles, any activity that engages the relaxation response can serve to quell catastrophizing and related distress. Treatments that evoke the relaxation response include diaphragmatic breathing, progressive muscle relaxation, hypnosis, mindfulness meditation, exercise, and yoga (see Chapter 5).

Pain Catastrophizing Undermines Pain Treatment Response

Pain catastrophizing is also associated with poor response to various pain treatments, including surgery and multidisciplinary pain treatment. In other words, catastrophizing appears to undermine results for many of the pain treatments doctors may try (Burns, Glenn, et al., 2003; Burns, Kubilus, Bruehl, Harden, & Lofland, 2003; Rosenberg, Schultz, Duarte, Rosen, & Raza, 2015; Vissers et al., 2012; Wertli et al., 2014)—thereby contributing to overmedicalization and possibly further despair and helplessness about pain. Pain catastrophizing amplifies pain processing in the brain and spinal cord (Gracely et al., 2004; Seminowicz & Davis, 2006). In addition, feelings of helplessness about pain may impede engagement in activity and movement therapies, thereby maintaining cycles of disability (M. J. L. Sullivan, Lynch, & Clark, 2005). Evidence-based psychological and behavioral treatment for pain allows patients to understand what they can do to help themselves feel better, regain control, and engage in self-management practices that will gain them long-term improvements. Pain catastrophizing illustrates why supportive counseling is insufficient for effectively addressing the psychological contribution to chronic pain. Simply describing one's challenges does not in itself lead to productive behavior change and may contribute to increased despair about pain. Pain education and specific skills must be learned and used daily to self-regulate distress, entrain adaptive neural patterns, and create positive patterns of behavior that enhance self-efficacy—and give medical treatments the best chance of working.

Researchers have shown that if pain catastrophizing is reduced early on in multidisciplinary treatment, the result is an improved overall response to multidisciplinary pain care, with better pain control and reduced pain interference with daily activities (Burns, Day, & Thorn, 2012). Results from fibromyalgia research have similarly shown that reducing pain catastrophizing early on leads to later reductions in fibromyalgia pain (Finan et al., 2013).

Carlos's Story

Carlos and his wife, Maria, had been married for 16 years.[1] Maria had multiple sclerosis, and Carlos helped her with many activities of daily living and took care of their home. Recently, Carlos developed excruciating facial pain. Although the pain was bad enough, he found himself feeling terrified and helpless a lot. He was used to being the caregiver, not the patient! So far, his doctor had been unable to help him. What if he was left with this much pain forever? Who would care for Maria? Who would take care of him? He found himself stuck in cycles of fear, depression, and pain. Several times during these cycles his pain became unbearable, and he went to the hospital emergency room for treatment. The first few times the doctors gave him strong opioids which reduced his pain and helped him calm down—temporarily. But the next day his fear about his

---

[1]The case example used in this chapter is fictitious or has been disguised to protect confidentiality.

pain and his and Maria's future would return and take over his thoughts and his attention.

Carlos's story illustrates how pain catastrophizing can negatively affect pain and pain treatment needs. Carlos's distress about his pain was clearly amplifying his pain. He had no skills or techniques to calm himself and therefore was reliant on medications to do it for him—a bad set up. In working with a pain psychologist, Carlos was able to learn about pain catastrophizing and why it is important to treat it. He learned how to identify his catastrophizing thoughts and how he could stop them in the moment. Carlos learned several pain-CBT techniques, including cognitive reframing and distraction, both of which helped him stop ruminating and magnifying his pain. He learned skills to calm his nervous system, and using these regularly helped quell his anxiety and his pain. Rather than expending all his energy on fearing the worst-case scenario, Carlos began focusing on what he could do to help himself and Maria. Carlos worked with a psychologist individually, and he also took an 8-week pain-CBT class where he was comforted by feeling understood and supported by peers who were also challenged by pain. He was inspired to learn from others and was excited to learn that through the journey he had much to offer others as well.

Additional Considerations: Healthy Individuals, Surgery, and Pediatrics

Healthy Individuals

Healthy individuals with higher PCS scores are 1.7 times more likely to develop chronic back pain following an acute back pain episode, whereas low PCS scores indicate a greater likelihood of having back pain resolved (Picavet, Vlaeyen, & Schouten, 2002). This means that pain catastrophizing is universally relevant because it can predict future pain, disease, and health.

Catastrophizing and Surgery

Research shows that individuals with higher PCS scores before surgery have poorer surgical outcomes, even controlling for medical and surgical factors. In fact, some research has suggested that pain catastrophizing is a better predictor of surgical outcomes than the surgery type, the surgeon, or disease characteristics, thereby underscoring the importance of optimizing psychobehavioral factors before surgery whenever possible (Theunissen, Peters, Bruce, Gramke, & Marcus, 2012). Prospective research has linked greater pain catastrophizing to longer hospital stays (Witvrouw et al., 2009), greater pain intensity after surgery (Pavlin, Sullivan, Freund, & Roesen, 2005; Vranceanu et al., 2010), greater use of opioids (Helmerhorst et al., 2014), delayed functional recovery (Roh et al., 2014), and greater likelihood to experience postsurgical chronic pain (Riddle, Wade, Jiranek, & Kong, 2010).

Pediatric Pain Catastrophizing

Although the focus of this text is on adult chronic pain, pediatric pain catastrophizing bears brief mention here. Pediatric chronic pain is complex because it involves more than just the child or teen; it also involves the parent(s) or caregiver(s). As such, it is insufficient only to measure whether children are catastrophizing their pain. Equally important is whether a parent or caregiver is catastrophizing the child's pain.

For child chronic pain, catastrophizing must be assessed two ways:

(a) Is the child catastrophizing his or her pain?
(b) Is the parent catastrophizing his or her child's pain?

Chronic pain affects 15% to 30% of children, and the cause of pain is often unknown (Friedrichsdorf et al., 2016). Seeing one's child in pain and distress, searching unsuccessfully for medical answers, feeling helpless to take the pain away, and experiencing increasing medical costs can all contribute to mounting stress in parents, an ever-growing anxious desire for the child's pain to go away and an increasing sense of helplessness that they cannot fix their child's discomfort and distress.

Despite parent catastrophizing generally coming from well-intentioned concern, it is known to have unintended detrimental effects on the child.

Parental catastrophizing may become a self-fulfilling prophecy for child pain. Parents' protective efforts to help their child's pain can boomerang and lead to greater disability (Wilson, Moss, Palermo, & Fales, 2014), sick days from school (Logan, Simons, & Carpino, 2012), and greater pain. Parents who catastrophize their child's pain may enable them to withdraw from their usual activities, thereby unwittingly shaping their child's behavior toward adoption of the "sick role." Although it is rarely conscious behavior on the part of parents, subtly or overtly encouraging sick role behaviors may prevent children from engaging in activities that would facilitate rehabilitation and help them to become more active in spite of their pain. A final consideration is that the children of parents with chronic pain are at increased risk to develop chronic pain themselves. Although some of the risk may involve genetic factors, the environment also plays a powerful role (Wilson et al., 2014). Parental chronic pain may shape aspects of the development and experience of child pain through modeling and learned behaviors. Adaptive pain management practices are important for the parent who has chronic pain; these serve as important adaptive modeling for children during the critical formative years when their health and health behaviors are being established.

PAIN-RELATED ANXIETY, FEAR OF PAIN, AND KINESIOPHOBIA

Like catastrophizing, pain-related anxiety and fear of pain are important considerations in chronic pain because they enhance the threat value of pain and, therefore, pain itself. Prospective studies have shown that fear of pain predicts the development of new-onset back pain 1 year after a pain-free baseline (Linton, Buer, Vlaeyen, & Hellsing, 2000). Similarly, kinesiophobia or fear of movement has been prospectively associated with the development of future back pain in population studies (Picavet et al., 2002). Pain-related anxiety and fear of pain may shape avoidance behavior and facilitate disability (Gheldof et al., 2010; Vlaeyen & Crombez, 1999; Vlaeyen, Crombez, & Linton, 2016). The fear-avoidance model posits that activity avoidance may contribute to physical changes (e.g., muscle tension, disuse, and atrophy) that may promote greater pain upon movement—therefore confirming the patient's underlying fear-related bias (Vlaeyen & Crombez, 1999; Vlaeyen et al., 2016). Pain-CBT and graded exposure therapy may effectively address these psychobehavioral factors, as can physical therapy with a therapist skilled in treating chronic pain (George, Fritz, Bialosky, & Donald, 2003; George, Wittmer, Fillingim, & Robinson, 2010; Woods & Asmundson, 2008). Treatment typically includes engaging patients in a graded exposure to therapeutic movement and exercises. The goals are to help patients (a) slowly begin appropriate movement, (b) gain strength and endurance, (c) challenge and extinguish maladaptive pain beliefs and fear of movement and/or pain and catastrophizing, (d) reduce avoidance behaviors, (e) understand that movement is vital to recovery of function, (f) increase self-efficacy for activity, (g) reduce pain-related interference and disability, and (h) actively engage in a daily pain self-management plan. Addressing pain-specific psychobehavioral factors is crucial for helping patients develop *pain self-efficacy*—confidence that they can engage in activities in spite of their pain. Often there is an underlying belief that pain equals harm (discussed further in Chapter 4), and this can be effectively addressed with proper pain science education (see *Explain Pain* by Butler and Moseley and other resources at the end of this chapter). Graded exposure to the feared movements—often coupled with relaxation—often reduces anxiety and fears and facilitates the cultivation of self-efficacy to manage distress and movement in the context of pain successfully. Patients begin to adopt an active role in the management of their pain and health. Through better engagement in activities and therapeutic exercises, patients can restore functioning and gain control over their chronic pain.

Pain-specific psychobehavioral factors are evaluated most often within the context of a specialty pain psychology evaluation. However, all mental health professionals can play a role in assessment and treatment, even if only to educate patients and refer them to pain specialists. Existing pain-specific resources may be a valuable addition to your clinical toolbox; such pain resources may be integrated into the therapy sessions and/or assigned as home reading and exercises.

KEY POINTS

- Pain catastrophizing is associated with greater pain, disability, and ongoing health problems.
- Pain catastrophizing undermines response to medical treatments for pain.
- Pain catastrophizing amplifies pain processing in the brain and spinal cord. Over time, brain structure and function are shaped toward greater pain and distress.
- Pain-specific psychobehavioral factors (fear of pain, pain anxiety, kinesiophobia, and pain catastrophizing) impede active engagement in rehabilitation and contribute to the persistence of pain.
- Pain education can treat maladaptive pain beliefs and behavioral patterns.
- CBT can help patients gain pain self-efficacy as function improves through active self-management.
- The term "pain catastrophizing" may be perceived negatively by some patients. "Negative pain mind-set" can serve as a useful replacement term for clinical conversations.

RESOURCES

Pain Catastrophizing Clinician Manual

The Pain Catastrophizing Scale User Manual (with cited scientific background):

Sullivan, M. J. L. (2009). *The Pain Catastrophizing Scale user manual.* Retrieved from http://sullivan-painresearch.mcgill.ca/pdf/pcs/PCSManual_English.pdf

Books

Pain science book:

Butler, D., & Moseley, G. L. (2003). *Explain pain.* Adelaide, Australia: Noigroup.

Patient books that specifically address catastrophizing:

Darnall, B. (2014). *Less pain, fewer pills: Avoid the dangers of prescription opioids and gain control over chronic pain.* Boulder, CO: Bull Publishing Company.

Darnall, B. (2016). *The opioid-free pain relief kit: 10 simple steps to ease your pain.* Boulder, CO: Bull Publishing Company.

Turk, D. W., & Winter F. (2006). *The pain survival guide: How to reclaim your life.* Washington, DC: American Psychological Association.

Videos

Darnall, B. [Stanford Pain Medicine]. (2015, August 3). *Stanford's Beth Darnall, PhD on pain catastrophizing* [Video file]. Retrieved from https://www.youtube.com/watch?v=fnNAF4EPFzc

GP Access and Hunter Integrated Pain Service [Painaustralia]. (2012, July 16). *Understanding pain: What to do about it in less than five minutes* [Video file]. Retrieved from https://www.youtube.com/watch?v=RWMKucuejIs

Work Wellness and Disability Prevention Institute. (2017, May 17). *Reducing catastrophizing to prevent and treat chronic pain* [Webinar]. Retrieved from http://cirpd.org/Webinars/Pages/Webinar.aspx?wbID=151

Pediatric Chronic Pain

Palermo, T. M., Valrie, C. R., & Carlson, C. W. (2014). Family and parent influences on pediatric chronic pain. *American Psychologist, 69,* 142–152. http://dx.doi.org/10.1037/a0035216

5

Overview of Evidence-Based Psychobehavioral Interventions for Pain

P ain research studies typically adhere to defined or manualized treatment protocols. But in real-world practice, the lines between psychological treatment modalities often blur as mental health therapists adapt their approach to meet the needs of the individual patient. For instance, my clinical training was cognitive behavioral, and my later training included mindfulness meditation. With years of clinical practice, I naturally evolved and integrated some key aspects of psychological flexibility—basic principles of acceptance and commitment therapy (ACT)—though I had no formalized training in ACT. Clinicians with diverse therapeutic approaches can be flexible and adapt to a patient's specific needs. And as such, they are equipped to help patients develop a tool kit of diverse self-regulatory skills.

All psychological treatments for pain share a goal of improving self-regulation. All psychological treatment approaches offer somewhat

http://dx.doi.org/10.1037/0000104-006
Psychological Treatment for Patients With Chronic Pain, by B. D. Darnall

---

PSYCHOBEHAVIORAL TREATMENTS FOR CHRONIC PAIN

- Cognitive behavioral therapy for pain
- Acceptance and commitment therapy
- Mindfulness-based stress reduction
- Meditation
- Hypnosis
- Biofeedback
- Chronic pain self-management

---

different pathways to improved self-regulation of thoughts, emotions, and/or physiological responses to pain and stress. Table 5.1 illustrates some of the similarities and distinctions between the various treatments discussed in detail in the next three chapters. Note that the selected components of the treatment list are not exhaustive. Pain education is one element of treatment that is unique to pain-specific psychological approaches, and the relaxation response is an element that is common to all psychological treatment approaches.

PAIN EDUCATION

Education about pain is an important component of pain-specific psychological treatments, such as cognitive behavioral therapy for pain (pain-CBT), ACT, and chronic pain self-management programs. Basic pain education helps patients better understand their experience, and it serves to challenge many false beliefs—such as "hurt equals harm" or "my life is over because I have chronic pain"—that can contribute to fear-avoidance behavior, disability, and amplified pain.

Pain education typically includes content similar to the first few chapters of this book: distinguishing between acute and chronic pain, individual factors that influence pain intensity, and the role of psychological factors and self-management behaviors in improving function

Table 5.1

Psychobehavioral Treatments for Chronic Pain

Selected components of treatment	Treatment type						
	Pain-CBT	Pain-ACT	MBSR	Meditation	Hypnosis	Biofeed-back	Pain self-management
Pain education	x	x				x	x
Cognitive reframing	x						
Nonreaction to thought		x	x	x			
Relaxation response	x	x	x	x	x	x	x
Visualization					x		
Problem-solving	x	x					x
Exercise goal	x	x					x
Action planning	x	x					x
Skills practice mastery	x	x	x	x	x	x	x

Note. MBSR = mindfulness-based stress reduction; Pain-ACT = acceptance and commitment therapy for pain; Pain-CBT = cognitive behavioral therapy for pain.

and reducing suffering from pain. Often pain education underscores the importance of activity goal setting and gradually increasing activity as a critical component of pain management and as a pathway to reducing pain interference and improving function, goal attainment, and quality of life.

Studies have shown that greater knowledge about pain neuroscience or pain neurophysiology is associated with reduced fear-avoidance behavior and perceived disability (Fletcher, Bradnam, & Barr, 2016). Providing proper education about pain is an effective intervention on its own.

THE RELAXATION RESPONSE

The relaxation response is a central component of all psychological treatments for pain, even those that are not pain specific. Pain treatments such as CBT, ACT, and self-management all include information about the relaxation response and its role in pain management. The relaxation response is also an indirect component of other pain treatments that include diaphragmatic breathing but may not specifically address pain, such as meditation.

The Relaxation Response Calms the Nervous System

Heart rate, respiratory rate, and skin temperature are automatically controlled by the sympathetic nervous system. Pain activates the sympathetic nervous system and automatically causes changes in breathing, blood pressure, skin temperature, and muscle tension. These changes can promote heightened stress, anxiety, and even greater pain. For these reasons, it is important for patients to learn ways to counteract the way the body naturally responds to pain. In doing so, individuals gain better control over their bodies, and in turn, self-efficacy is enhanced and pain relief is gained.

The relaxation response is a useful tool for decreasing pain-related distress and for disrupting catastrophizing thought patterns. In addition, it is often combined with a body scan so patients can learn to read their body cues early on, pace their activities according to the cues they observe, and deliver better self-care. Patients learn to use the relaxation response regularly to calm their nervous system and in doing so can begin to self-regulate responses to pain, including the physiologic, cognitive, and emotion response patterns that may be counterproductively worsening their pain. The relaxation response is an important tool to help patients increase and master self-regulation in the context of pain (Metikaridis, Hadjipavlou, Artemiadis, Chrousos, & Darviri, 2016). In addition to increasing self-efficacy for controlling pain and pain-related distress, improved self-regulation helps lower stress-related activity in the hypothalamic–pituitary–adrenal axis and the immune system, thereby promoting better mental and physical health (Steptoe, Hamer, & Chida, 2007).

The Relaxation Response Dually Targets the Effects of Stress and Pain

Stress and pain activate the sympathetic nervous system and trigger the same physiological cascade that includes increased heart rate and respiratory rate and muscle and blood vessel constriction and can facilitate a mental focus on the stressor. Because pain and stress share neurobiological cause and effect, they are bidirectionally related. Living with chronic pain is stressful, and most individuals note that stress amplifies their pain and reduces their ability to cope effectively, though few understand the shared neurobiology.

> Stress and pain activate the sympathetic nervous system and trigger the same physiological cascade. Chronic pain leads to ongoing, automatic physiological responses that entrain the brain and body toward greater pain.

Although the job of the sympathetic nervous system is to activate the fight-or-flight response that enhances survival by equipping one to escape the threat of harm, persistent activation of the sympathetic nervous system only primes a person to have greater pain. A critical part of chronic pain management is helping patients learn ways to counteract their hardwired pain responses (sympathetic nervous system activation) by instead activating the parasympathetic nervous system (e.g., via the relaxation response; see Table 5.2 for a comparison of sympathetic nervous system vs. parasympathetic nervous system responses). Activation of the parasympathetic nervous system helps train mind and body away from pain, giving patients a critical level of control over pain and suffering.

The relaxation response is physiological and measurable. Biofeedback is a tool that is used to demonstrate to patients the physiological effects

Table 5.2
Components of Various Psychobehavioral Treatments for Pain

Sympathetic nervous system activation	Parasympathetic nervous system activation
Rapid heart rate	Slowed heart rate
Short, shallow breathing	Deep, diaphragmatic breathing
Vasoconstriction	Vasodilation
Increased cortisol	Normalized cortisol
Increased adrenaline	Normalized adrenaline
Anxious, fearful	Calm, peaceful
Causes or triggers	
Automatic responses to pain, stress	Relaxation response
	• Diaphragmatic breathing
	• Meditation
	• Exercise

that the relaxation response has on heart rate, respiratory rate, muscle tension, and skin temperature (see Chapter 7 for more on biofeedback). Despite its clear biological effects, studies have suggested that the benefits of the relaxation response are mainly due to its psychological effects. As patients gain mastery with relaxation skills, they cultivate positive beliefs and confidence in their control over pain (self-efficacy), which then leads to pain and stress relief.

SONIA'S STORY

Sonia had a fender bender 6 months ago.[1] Her car was fine, but she had had frequent headaches ever since. She was on edge a lot, and like most people, she carried a lot of tension in her neck and shoulders. The problem was that this tension was causing her tension headaches to flare. The more pain she had, the more tense she became—it was a vicious cycle, and she felt at its mercy. Sonia found a psychologist who

---

[1]The case example used in this chapter is fictitious or has been disguised to protect confidentiality.

understood how to help her. Sonia learned about how pain affects the whole person, from the muscles to the nervous system to emotions and even to daily choices. She learned that she had to begin shaping her brain and body away from pain and that the relaxation response could help her do that. At first, she was skeptical, but after trying a guided exercise in session, her pre–post stress and muscle tension ratings gave her all the evidence she needed. She was more relaxed, and her neck was less tense. She set a goal of practicing the relaxation response several times daily to retrain her neuromuscular patterns and to induce overall pain-relieving calm. She felt great after each practice, but then the tension would creep back in after about a half hour or so—this was expected. After about a month of regular practice, she noticed that her overall tension levels were lower, and she was generally calmer. Her real progress was noted in her headache log: She was having fewer headache days per week, and even when she had headaches, they were less intense and less impactful. She was excited to learn that she was in control, and she resolved to do everything she could to maintain control.

KEY POINTS

- All evidence-based psychological treatment for pain involves activating the relaxation response and use of skills that directly or indirectly promote regulation of cognition, emotion, and physiological arousal.
- Pain education is an effective psychological intervention that can challenge maladaptive pain beliefs about the meaning of pain. Pain-CBT, pain-ACT, and chronic pain self-management include pain education.

RESOURCES[2]

Pain Education Book

Butler, D., & Moseley, G. L. (2003). *Explain pain.* Adelaide, Australia: Noigroup.

---

[2]Try the tools and materials you will be recommending to your patients. By doing so, you become equipped to explain their value and have follow-up discussions with your patients about what they are learning and how they are applying the various skills.

Relaxation Response Tools

Free mobile relaxation app (from the U.S. Department of Defense):

National Center for Telehealth & Technology. (2016). Breathe2Relax (Version 1.7) [Mobile application software]. Retrieved from http://t2health.dcoe.mil/ apps/breathe2relax

Binaural audio file (CD or MP3; 20 minutes) includes diaphragmatic breathing, progressive muscle relaxation, and autogenic training (https:// www.bullpub.com/catalog/EPM):

Darnall, B. (2014). Enhanced pain management [Audio CD or MP3]. Boulder, CO: Bull Publishing Company.

Articles

An overview of psychological treatments for chronic pain:

Sturgeon, J. A. (2014). Psychological therapies for the management of chronic pain. *Psychology Research and Behavior Management*, *7*, 115–124. http:// dx.doi.org/10.2147/PRBM.S44762

Psychological treatments and pain neurophysiology (open access):

Flor, H. (2014). Psychological pain intervention and neurophysiology: Implications for a mechanism-based approach. *American Psychologist*, *69*, 188–196. Retrieved from http://www.apa.org/pubs/journals/releases/amp-a0035254.pdf

6

Cognitive Behavioral Therapy and Acceptance and Commitment Therapy for Chronic Pain

Cognitive behavioral therapy for pain (pain-CBT) has roughly 30 years of scientific evidence to support its efficacy in across a variety of chronic pain conditions. Pain-CBT is similar to CBT for psychological conditions but is highly tailored to meet the specific needs of individuals with chronic pain. Specific tailoring involves content on pain education; the connection between mood and pain; the connection between thoughts, emotions, and pain; activity pacing within the context of pain; addressing maladaptive pain beliefs and pain catastrophizing; reducing pain behaviors; setting appropriate activity goals and gradually increasing activity; and increasing general wellness and self-care behaviors. In short, the pain-CBT protocol is centered on the self-management of chronic pain, including related distress. For this reason, general CBT delivered to a patient with chronic pain does not equal pain-CBT. Pain-CBT specifically addresses pain-related psychobehavioral factors and requires mental

http://dx.doi.org/10.1037/0000104-007
Psychological Treatment for Patients With Chronic Pain, by B. D. Darnall

health professionals to have training in these areas and/or follow a manualized protocol (see the pain-CBT resources at the end of this chapter).

Table 6.1 illustrates the distinctions between pain-CBT and CBT for
depression. The table also provides a general guide to topics covered in
pain-CBT.

Pain-CBT is considered the gold-standard psychological treatment
for chronic pain because it has the best evidence to support its effectiveness across a variety of chronic pain conditions. It is worth noting that
pain-CBT has been studied for 3 decades, whereas other pain treatment
approaches may be newer or less studied in the context of pain. The goals
of pain-CBT are to reduce pain and psychological distress and to improve
physical and role function by decreasing unhelpful pain beliefs and
behaviors, increasing wellness behaviors, and enhancing self-regulation

Table 6.1

Comparison of Content in Cognitive Behavioral Therapy for Pain Versus Cognitive Behavioral Therapy for Depression

Content/topics	Pain-CBT	CBT for depression
Pain education	x	
Activity pacing	x	
Pain catastrophizing	x	
Pain beliefs	x	
Cognitive reframing	x Specific to pain	x
Relaxation training	x	x
Mood regulation	x Specific to pain	x
Problem-solving	x Specific to pain	x
Sleep hygiene	x	x
Exercise and movement	x	x
Goal setting	x	x

Note. CBT = cognitive behavioral therapy.

and self-management of pain overall (Ehde, Dillworth, & Turner, 2014). Research has shown that pain-CBT improves positive adaptation, mood, and function by reducing pain behaviors and fear avoidance, as well as catastrophic thinking related to pain. As outlined in Chapters 3 and 4, these are important therapeutic targets for pain-CBT because they associate with greater pain disability, greater pain intensity, depression, and activity limitations. Pain-CBT guides patients to identify maladaptive pain beliefs and thoughts and extinguish negative thoughts with cognitive reframing, positive distraction, or application of relaxation skills. Cognitively, patients learn to monitor and evaluate their thoughts with respect to how adaptive (e.g., reassuring, calming) or maladaptive (e.g., alarming, distressing) they are and to develop adaptive thoughts and use them to decrease distress about pain or other factors (Sturgeon, 2014). Behaviorally, patients are guided toward active goal setting, appropriate activation and activity pacing, a gradual increase in activity and exercise over time, increasing social and pleasant activities, and improved self-care.

Table 6.2 illustrates the relationship between common pain beliefs, behavioral responses, and negative results and illustrates the importance of dismantling maladaptive pain beliefs to optimize function, pain relief, and overall mental and physical well-being.

A trained psychologist delivers pain-CBT to individual patients or groups of patients with chronic pain. Most of the pain-CBT research has reported findings for studies that use manualized, group treatment protocols involving eight to 10 weekly sessions lasting about 2 hours each. An appealing aspect of group pain-CBT is the social dynamic. Patients learn from each other and support one another, and group treatment can be particularly beneficial for those who are socially isolated. Group pain-CBT incorporates into each session interactive discussion, practice of relaxation training, action planning, and home exercises. In essence, participants learn how best to alleviate their pain and symptoms while moving toward achieving the goals that matter to them.

Pain-CBT has been shown to be effective for reducing pain intensity, pain catastrophizing, depression, and social impacts (Stewart et al., 2015); a meta-analysis in back pain found similar results (Hoffman, Papas,

Table 6.2

Common Pain Beliefs, Typical Behavioral Responses, and Outcomes

Common pain belief	Behavioral response	Result
"If I move less my pain is better."	Patient becomes sedentary, deactivated, and deconditioned.	Over time, deactivation and deconditioning worsen pain and may lead to onset of new pain problems. Mood and sleep may deteriorate.
"If I can just fix my pain I will get my life back." Also: "I have a diagnosis; my pain is a medical problem."	Overly focused on a medical "cure." Delayed engagement in rehabilitation and self-management approaches that gain best results for function and relief. Putting life on hold; making activities contingent on pain.	External locus of control. Feeling at the mercy of pain or a victim of the situation. Overreliance on medical system, doctors, pills, and procedures that are of limited value without psychology and movement therapies. Poor results for desired pain relief.
Pain equals harm.	Fear of pain, catastrophizing, and fear of movement (kinesiophobia) may develop and increase.	Stopping activities and rehabilitative processes. Deactivation. Amplified pain from catastrophizing.

Chatkoff, & Kerns, 2007). Another meta-analysis considered a broad array of pain types and found that pain-CBT was most effective for reducing depression and pain catastrophizing (moderate effects), though it is noted to have small effects for pain and disability (Williams, Eccleston, & Morley, 2012).

COGNITIVE BEHAVIORAL THERAPY FOR PAIN CHANGES THE BRAIN

Neuroimaging research using magnetic resonance imaging brain scans before and after an 11-week group pain-CBT yielded striking results. Researchers reported that the pretreatment brain scans of patients with chronic pain showed gray matter volumetric decreases in the prefrontal

> Pain-CBT has been shown to increase volume in the regions of the brain associated with pain control.

context and somatosensory regions of the brain associated with pain control (Seminowicz et al., 2013). After pain-CBT, patient scans evidenced significant volumetric increases in those same brain regions, and results correlated with patient reports of pain relief. Furthermore, the researchers found that these increases were fully mediated by reductions in pain catastrophizing, further underscoring the need to identify and treat pain catastrophizing as a pathway to psychobiobehavioral recovery from pain. Patient receptivity to psychological treatment for pain may be enhanced by sharing these scientific findings that evidence a biological mechanism for psychological treatment success. Other research has shown that 12 weeks of pain-CBT led to normalization of abnormal intrinsic connectivity in resting-state brain networks, and this was associated with reduced pain intensity (Yoshino et al., 2018). Sharing the science of pain psychology treatment may facilitate patient engagement in pain-CBT and other treatment modalities. Lasting changes in brain structure and function suggest enduring brain effects, though long-term studies are needed.

Some studies have suggested that the self-reported benefits of pain-CBT are sustained at 1-year follow-up (Turner et al., 2016), whereas others have suggested some decay of effects at 6-month follow-up. Patients should be periodically assessed to determine whether an additional course of pain-CBT treatment may be indicated, whether a few booster sessions can address any relapse effects, or whether additional treatment modalities may be indicated (e.g., mindfulness-based stress reduction, acceptance and commitment therapy). Pain-CBT provides individuals with the road map and skills to manage their pain, but they may require ongoing supportive structure and coaching to maintain behaviors until they become ingrained. Individual results are predicated on the daily, regular use of the skills and their commitment to good pain management principles. All mental health professionals can help their clients adopt a self-management mind-set for chronic pain. Like diabetes or any other health condition, managing pain must become and remain a daily priority. As such, the journey does not end after 8 weeks of pain-CBT; rather, the journey is just beginning.

LUCA'S STORY OF COGNITIVE BEHAVIORAL THERAPY FOR PAIN

Luca had fibromyalgia and chronic fatigue.[1] His pain and fatigue waxed and waned. When he finally hit that sweet spot of relatively low pain and decent energy, he felt great pressure to accomplish all the tasks he had been neglecting for days or weeks. He would be highly productive for a few hours before hitting a wall of pain and exhaustion. Typically, he would need days to recover from the pain flare. His doctor referred him to group pain-CBT so he could learn ways to self-manage his chronic pain. Luca learned many things in pain-CBT, but three points stood out for him. First, he learned that he had to set realistic expectations. Over time he lost sight of what was realistic—he was focusing on what he wanted to do versus what he was truly capable of doing without flaring his pain. Learning to distinguish the two and set appropriate activity goals that honored his body's limits was key. Second, he learned that he could avoid many pain flares with good activity pacing principles. Instead of pushing 100% when he felt good, he learned to keep a gentle, steady pace all the time. In doing so, he stopped making his activity contingent on his pain and started learning to live life every single day. By not pushing so hard on good days he found he could extend them much longer, and that helped his pain and his mood. Third, he learned that he was pushing himself so hard because he feared losing control if he did not push himself. It was through the group he began to see that his attempts to gain control were doing the opposite by increasing his pain. Luca began learning to adjust his expectations, and in doing so, he learned to be gentle with himself and take better care of himself. Instead of punishing himself when he felt

---

[1]The case examples used in this chapter are fictitious or have been disguised to protect confidentiality.

good, he learned to savor these times and extend them with good self-management practices.

ACCEPTANCE AND COMMITMENT THERAPY

Acceptance and commitment therapy (ACT) is also referred to as *contextual CBT*. Although pain-CBT includes content on identifying and altering maladaptive thought patterns, ACT does not. ACT promotes nonreactivity to negative thoughts as a way to diffuse them. ACT treatment for chronic pain guides acceptance of what is in one's life right now, mindfulness of one's values and goals, awareness of one's available choices, and commitment to oneself to do what will move one closer to attaining valued goals. ACT helps individuals clarify what is most meaningful to them and motivates personal, inspired change and a value-driven life. The combination of psychological and behavioral skills equips one to be less triggered and affected by negative thoughts, feelings, and experiences.

Whereas CBT includes thought evaluation and change, ACT theory posits that attempts to control or manage emotional processes can create problems and compound suffering. As such, ACT aligns with mindfulness principles to allow patients to develop a new and compassionate relationship with pain and other experiences. Patients are guided toward present-time, moment-to-moment, nonjudgmental awareness of their thoughts and full, flexible, nondefensive, nonreactive contact with experienced events. Rather than "fighting against pain," patients are guided to begin to develop positive, attainable goals that are consistent with their values. The focus of treatment is on enhancing psychological flexibility, nonreactivity to negative thoughts, and goal-directed behavior toward personally meaningful and valued goals. Importantly, ACT emphasizes engagement in activities with pain present, rather than waiting for the pain to subside.

The goal of ACT is not the elimination of difficult feelings; rather, it is to be present with what life brings and to move one toward valued behavior. ACT invites patients to open up to unpleasant feelings, to not overreact to them, and to not avoid situations in which they are experienced. Troublesome thoughts are not evaluated or disputed; rather, patients are guided to use a variety of techniques to diffuse them. Examples of thought diffusion techniques include observing negative thoughts dispassionately; repeating negative thoughts out loud until only their sound remains; treating thoughts as an external observation by giving them shape, size, color, speed, or form; thanking the mind for such an interesting thought, saying it slowly, or labeling the process of thinking (e.g., "I am having the thought that I cannot do anything because of pain").

A randomized controlled study for a 12-week ACT intervention in fibromyalgia suggested that ACT was effective for reducing pain-related disability and improving self-efficacy, depression, impact of fibromyalgia, and anxiety (Wicksell et al., 2013). The researchers reported that ACT-related improvements appeared to be mediated by increased psychological flexibility.

> Rather than seeking to change negative thoughts, ACT promotes mindful observation of thoughts as a way to diffuse their charge.

To date, ACT has not demonstrated superiority to CBT for chronic pain (Öst, 2014). However, ACT may be particularly suitable for patients who have perceptions of injustice and feel victimized by their pain, the circumstances that caused their pain condition, their medical care, or other life factors.

CARMEN'S STORY OF ACCEPTANCE AND COMMITMENT THERAPY

Carmen's life changed when she was diagnosed with Stage 3 cancer 2 years ago. She was immediately scheduled for radiation and chemotherapy and even had surgery to cut out a tumor. She had pain from the cancer, but after that was treated, she was dismayed that she had new kinds of severe pain that were caused by the cancer treatment. It was called neuropathic pain, and it was debilitating. Although she was happy to be in remission, she never got back on her feet and into life again. She could not deal with the pain and was trying many medications; those made her groggy, so she was not just in bed most of the day, now she was sleeping through most of the day. The worst part was that she was spending little time with her son and daughter, who were 5 and 7 years old. She felt guilty for being sick and absent from much of their daily lives, and she was angry at the medical system for creating these new problems that seemed unsolvable. The injustice of it was too much. She wanted her doctors to fix her pain so she could move forward, live normally, and be a good mother to her children.

Carmen's friend recommended she see her therapist, an ACT specialist. After several weeks, Carmen developed mindfulness skills to help anchor her in the present moment without reacting to it. She learned to identify her thought "triggers" and how she could use different language and techniques to lessen their negative impact. Overall, she was finding she was less reactive to her pain, and her anger was dissipating somewhat. Carmen was able to identify that her most important value was spending time with her family and being an engaged mom. She worked with her therapist to create goals that were consistent with these core values. Rather than waiting for her doctors to fix things—and feeling angry, stuck, and in bed all the time—she set goals and began taking small steps toward attaining a life that was consistent with her core values. She realized she was unlikely to be as active as her prepain self, but she began to see that she could still be engaged with her family and parent her children despite her pain. She was excited about the emotional freedom she felt, and releasing her anger and resentment allowed her to begin working more productively with her doctors too.

CHRONIC PAIN SELF-MANAGEMENT

At the core, all behavioral pain management approaches seek to equip patients with the ability to self-manage pain and symptoms. Beyond the concept of behavioral self-management of pain, there are formal treatment programs for chronic disease self-management. The Arthritis Self-Management Program, a program that revolves around managing pain, was started 40 years ago (Lorig, 1982; Lorig & Holman, 1993; Lorig, Lubeck, Kraines, Seleznick, & Holman, 1985; Lorig, Ritter, Laurent, & Fries, 2004; Marks & Allegrante, 2005). In recent years, the Chronic Pain Self-Management Program (CPSMP) was developed as a manualized group treatment pathway for chronic pain. CPSMP is an effective behavioral treatment, albeit backed by weaker evidence than exists for pain-CBT.

The CPSMP is an evidence-based group treatment and, uniquely, it is delivered by trained peer coleaders with lived experience in successful pain self-management (no other evidence pain treatments involve peer leaders). Peers are usually people with chronic pain who live in the communities in which they teach. Self-management is similar to pain-CBT in format and content, but because it is peer-led rather than psychologist led, it lacks content on cognitive restructuring. Like pain-CBT, CPSMP incorporates interactive discussion, practice of relaxation training, action planning, and home exercises into each session. Patients learn how to live better with chronic pain by making daily choices that support better health and function. CPSMP is most effective for improving pain self-efficacy across pain conditions (e.g., back pain, arthritis). Two peer coleaders (or trained professionals) provide patient education about pain and ways to effectively self-manage pain, its impacts, and other symptoms. Each 6-week workshop follows a highly structured manual, and content is delivered over six weekly 2-hour group sessions. Some patients may prefer CPSMP because it is peer led, and CPSMP may be a viable option in cases in which access to pain-CBT is limited. CPSMP is typically not covered by insurance—patients who receive care through a closed payer system should inquire about such services; many offer CPSMP free of charge. CPSMP is also offered free of charge through certain municipal health services and older adult wellness programs.

Courses are not typically covered by insurance but may be embedded into closed-payer networks (e.g., Intermountain Healthcare, Veterans Health Administration). In addition, many municipalities may offer self-management wellness courses through senior centers or other community services; the courses may be offered free of charge or fees may apply—be sure to check if costs exist. Self-management resources vary by region and community. To determine whether self-management courses exist in your area try the following steps:

1. Check first with your health care system or insurance carrier.
2. Google "chronic pain self-management" and your city to see whether courses exist there.

KEY POINTS

- Pain-CBT, pain-ACT, and chronic pain self-management include learning and applying problem-solving skills, activity pacing, and active goal setting.
- Pain-CBT has the most robust body of evidence to support its efficacy for chronic pain.
- Pain-ACT may be particularly beneficial for patients who have perceptions of injustice about their pain, disability, or other factors.

RESOURCES

Behavioral Health Therapist Locators

Acceptance and commitment therapy. Locate an ACT therapist anywhere in the world: https://contextualscience.org/civicrm/profile?gid=17&reset=1&force=1

Cognitive Behavioral Therapy for Pain

Free evidence-based treatment manual used by the Veterans Health Administration for CBT for pain:

Murphy, J. L., McKellar, J. D., Raffa, S. D., Clark, M. E., Kerns, R. D., Karlin, B. E. (2014). *Cognitive behavioral therapy for chronic pain: Therapist manual.* Retrieved from https://www.va.gov/PAINMANAGEMENT/docs/CBT-CP_Therapist_Manual.pdf

Free literacy-adapted CBT manuals for chronic pain. Beverly Thorn, PhD, has a wealth of resources available online, including a free pain-CBT workbook for clients as well as therapist scripts: http://pmt.ua.edu/publications.html

Mental Health Professional Books and Clinician Manuals

Group cognitive therapy for chronic pain instructional manual:

Thorn, B. E. (2017). *Cognitive therapy for chronic pain: A step-by-step guide* (2nd ed.). New York, NY: Guilford Press.

Therapist book for acceptance and commitment therapy:

Dahl, J., Wilson, K., Luciano, C., & Hayes, S. (2005). *Acceptance and commitment therapy for chronic pain.* Oakland, CA: Context Press.

Open Access Articles

CBT for chronic pain:

Ehde, D. M., Dillworth, T. M., & Turner, J. A. (2014). Cognitive behavioral therapy for individuals with chronic pain: Efficacy, innovations and directions for future research. *American Psychologist, 69,* 153–166. Retrieved from https://www.apa.org/pubs/journals/releases/amp-a0035747.pdf

ACT and mindfulness for chronic pain:

McCracken, L. M., & Vowles, K. E. (2014). Acceptance and commitment therapy and mindfulness for chronic pain: Model, process, and progress. *American Psychologist, 69,* 178–187. Retrieved from http://www.apa.org/pubs/journals/releases/amp-a0035623.pdf

Patient Books

CBT-based (workbook format):

Caudill, M. (2016). *Managing pain before it manages you.* New York, NY: Guilford Press.
Lewandowski, M. (2006). *The chronic pain care workbook.* Reno, NV: Lucky Bat Books.
Turk, D. W., & Winter, F. (2006). *The pain survival guide: How to reclaim your life.* Washington, DC: American Psychological Association.

Includes a guided, binaural relaxation audio file and CD:

Darnall, B. (2014). *Less pain, fewer pills: Avoid the dangers of prescription opioids and gain control over chronic pain.* Boulder, CO: Bull Publishing Company.

Includes a guided, binaural relaxation audio file:

Darnall, B. (2016). *The opioid-free pain relief kit: 10 simple steps to ease your pain.* Boulder, CO: Bull Publishing Company.

ACT for patients:

Dahl, J., Hayes, S. C., & Lundgren, T. (2006). *Living beyond your pain: Using acceptance and commitment therapy to ease chronic pain.* Oakland, CA: New Harbinger.

Video

Patient testimonial on CBT for chronic pain. In this brief video, a patient describes her successful experience with group CBT for chronic low-back pain:

Stanford Medicine [Stanford Pain Medicine]. (2017, June 25). *Tina CBT testimonial* [Video file]. Retrieved from http://bit.ly/cbtforchronicpain

CLINICAL TIPS FOR WORKING WITH CLIENTS WITH CHRONIC PAIN

- Validate the experience of pain. All pain is real, regardless of the medical diagnosis or lack thereof.
- Provide basic education about the role of psychology in the experience and treatment of pain.
- Everyone can benefit from psychological treatment for pain. The goal is to optimize control over pain and to improve function while needing less medical intervention.
- Online or in-person chronic pain support groups can help reduce social isolation and increase patient activity and engagement in their care. Learn about local supportive resources, then educate and encourage your patients to participate in them.

- Which treatment is best for my patient? For any patient, the best psychological treatment strategy is the one in which they are most likely to engage. All things being equal, the best evidence exists for pain-CBT (or a variant, such as ACT for chronic pain). Consider explaining the differences between the various treatment approaches and ask about individual preferences. Most patients have an opinion and appreciate a shared-decision approach. I usually recommend more than one approach. Exposure to a variety of pain management approaches allows patients to determine what works best for them, and it helps them acquire a broad tool kit of skills.
- Multiple pain psychology treatment pathways may yield best results due to
  - the extended nature of treatment if treatments are accessed sequentially,
  - ongoing social support associated with group treatments,
  - reinforcing messages about key pain management concepts,
  - diverse skill sets acquired across multiple treatment approaches, and
  - physical function and active engagement in functional goals promoted by ongoing appointments, particularly for clients who may be largely homebound or isolated.
- Group treatment may be contraindicated for psychological reasons (e.g., personality disorder or social anxiety disorder) or client preference.

7

Mindfulness Interventions, Hypnosis, and Biofeedback

This chapter discusses mindfulness interventions as evidence-based approaches to treating pain, as well as two important evidence-based procedures that treat pain: hypnosis and biofeedback.

MINDFULNESS INTERVENTIONS

Mindfulness interventions are rooted in Eastern philosophy and Buddhist tradition. Modern mindfulness interventions are typically secular—meaning that they have no religious affiliation. Mindfulness interventions are useful for bringing awareness to one's thoughts and present experience. The goal is to maintain awareness of the present moment while maintaining nonreactivity. In doing so, mindfulness practitioners gain relief from distress because they no longer perseverate on the past or continue to worry about the future. One learns to observe pain or thoughts about pain without attaching meaning or judgment to them.

http://dx.doi.org/10.1037/0000104-008
Psychological Treatment for Patients With Chronic Pain, by B. D. Darnall

Mindfulness-Based Stress Reduction

Mindfulness-based stress reduction (MBSR) is a structured treatment protocol that is rooted in mindfulness principles and practice. MBSR involves eight weekly 2-hour class sessions plus a daylong retreat. Participants cultivate mindful awareness through exercises that include mindful eating, mindful breathing, body scanning, changing the way one responds to discomfort, cultivating an openness to experience, and cultivating stress hardiness. MBSR includes education on stress and the mind–body connection. Participants gain an understanding of how to reduce reactivity to negative physical and emotional experiences, thereby disarming their charge and impact.

For chronic pain, research has suggested that MBSR effectively reduces pain catastrophizing, negative focus on somatic cues, and rumination. A recent randomized controlled trial that compared MBSR with cognitive behavioral therapy for pain (pain-CBT) in chronic low back pain showed equivalence between the two interventions for back pain and functional limitations at 6-month follow-up and for sustained reductions in catastrophizing at 1 year (Cherkin et al., 2016; Turner et al., 2016). Because MBSR is a general health and wellness intervention, it may be particularly suitable for individuals who have resistance to "psychological treatment" for chronic pain.

Special considerations exist for MBSR. It is taught by certified MBSR practitioners, and training in psychology is not required. MBSR is not typically covered by insurance, so costs are incurred as out-of-pocket expenses to patients. Though in-person MBSR treatment is best, the typical course fees of about $325 may be cost-prohibitive for many patients. See the end of the chapter for free resource options.

Mindfulness Meditation

Although MBSR is a highly structured course, mindfulness meditation is a technique that can be learned relatively quickly and can be used to reduce pain and distress. Mindfulness meditation helps control attention and direct attention away from pain. Often the beginning skill is diaphragmatic breathing and maintaining focus on the breath. If the mind wanders, one gently returns awareness to the breath, without judgment. Mindfulness meditation helps cultivate nonreactivity and an "observer" position over thoughts and circumstances. Like acceptance and commitment therapy (ACT), MBSR, and CBT-based relaxation training, mindfulness meditation allows individuals to quiet the mind and begin observing how mindful or diaphragmatic breathing can facilitate calmness.

In pain experiments conducted with healthy volunteers, brief mindfulness training was associated with a significant reduction in pain intensity and pain bothersomeness, and this was associated with neuroimaging findings of reducing pain processing in the brain (Zeidan et al., 2011). In short, mindfulness meditation appears to alter the way the brain functions, and it is associated with pain relief. It is important to note that used irregularly, techniques such as mindfulness meditation or diaphragmatic breathing confer immediate calming. However, it is the consistent, regular use of the skills and techniques that leads to enduring changes in the brain that correlate with patient reports of increased self-efficacy and longer term reductions in distress and pain.

HYPNOSIS

Hypnosis is a clinical procedure in which a trained psychologist typically conducts a relaxation induction, then suggests the patient experience changes in sensations, perceptions, thoughts or behavior. In the case of chronic pain, therapist suggestions are typically for relaxation, calmness, pleasure, and comfort. During hypnosis, the therapist may guide the patient to visualize pleasurable, safe, or comforting scenes and situations.

A meta-analysis of 18 hypnosis studies reported that 75% of clinical and experimental participants with different types of pain obtained pain relief from hypnotic techniques (Montgomery, DuHamel, & Redd, 2000). Hypnosis may benefit most people with chronic pain, though some patients are noted to be resistant to hypnosis.

Research has shown that hypnotic suggestion in patients with fibromyalgia effectively altered pain intensity, and this correlated with brain scan images showing altered pain processing activity (Derbyshire, Whalley, & Oakley, 2009).

BIOFEEDBACK

Chapter 5 describes the beneficial role of the relaxation response in activating the parasympathetic nervous system (PNS). The PNS counteracts how the brain and body respond to pain and stress (elevated heart rate, quick and shallow breathing, constricted blood vessels, muscle tension, anxiety or distress). These automatic pain and stress responses cause greater pain and distress, so it is important to learn ways to control them. As such, learning how to engage the PNS is an important pain management tool, and it is central to most evidence-based pain treatments. Diaphragmatic breathing, guided relaxation, and meditation are different ways to engage the relaxation response and PNS. In doing so, one can leverage mind and body away from pain. With regular skills use, patients gain mastery in their ability to counteract pain and stress, and they gain self-efficacy for pain management. And over time, individuals train mind and body to have an overall lower level of muscle tension and arousal, and this can offer a nice comfort buffer that allows them to be less reactive and negatively affected when pain and stress arise.

Biofeedback is a procedure that helps individuals learn how to engage their parasympathetic response and gain control over their pain and stress responses. Typically, biofeedback is performed by a certified biofeedback therapist or by a trained psychologist. Biofeedback involves using tools to measure indices of stress and pain. Electrodes are placed on various parts of the body to measure temperature, sweating, and heart rate. Electrodes are placed on the head, neck, shoulders, and other parts of the body to measure muscle tension. Certain types of biofeedback also measure neural (brain) activity (neurofeedback or electroencephalography). In all cases, the electrodes relay an individual's information to a computer. Biofeedback programs display the measurements on the monitor for the therapist and patient to see.

Biofeedback is dynamic and involves patients working to "change" their output numbers (indices of stress). Biofeedback therapists guide patients to learn that through diaphragmatic breathing and relaxation techniques, their output numbers get lower. Most programs make it fun and patient friendly. The numbers may be displayed as hot air balloons, and the goal is to help the hot air balloons land. Patients learn that by becoming relaxed, their balloons sink toward the ground. They also learn that using simple relaxation techniques can have a dramatic physiological response—their numbers prove it. Biofeedback provides patients with a skill set and understanding for why engaging the relaxation response (PNS) is important, and it can motivate them to include this powerful skill in their pain management tool kit.

It is important to note that biofeedback is simply a unique way of teaching the same skill set taught in pain-CBT, ACT, and generally in MBSR: the relaxation response. If patients are proficient with the relaxation response, they probably do not need biofeedback. Patients who are resistant to psychological treatments may be more receptive to biofeedback because of its clear emphasis on quantifying physiological output. Biofeedback can be a useful tool to help patients understand the power of the mind–body connection and how it affects chronic pain.

The pain-relieving effects of biofeedback have been demonstrated across a range of pain conditions, including back pain (Sielski, Rief, & Glombiewski, 2017), neck and shoulder pain (Ma et al., 2011), fibromyalgia (Glombiewski, Bernardy, & Häuser, 2013), temporomandibular joint disorders (TMJ; Crider, Glaros, & Gevirtz, 2005), and headache and migraine (Probyn et al., 2017). Biofeedback is particularly useful for pain conditions that are exacerbated by muscle tension, such as TMJ, tension headaches, and migraine. Research has suggested that biofeedback can be as or more effective for pain relief than medications and may serve as migraine prophylaxis (Probyn et al., 2017).

JAMES'S BIOFEEDBACK STORY

Like a lot of people, James had more than one type of chronic pain.[1] He had a degenerative hip condition and last year underwent hip replacement surgery. His hip pain improved some but not enough—he still rated

---

[1]The case example used in this chapter is fictitious or has been disguised to protect confidentiality.

his pain as 5/10 most days, and it was limiting his physical activities on a daily basis. The migraines were more episodic. He seemed to get about two to three migraines a month, and when one hit, everything stopped for at least a day, sometimes more. His doctor recommended he see a pain psychologist, but James was not interested in "mental health"—he wanted relief for his pain. His doctor knew that patients who were resistant to psychological treatment for pain were often more receptive to biofeedback, so she next suggested he see a biofeedback specialist for a few visits; James agreed. During his first session, James learned how to control his muscle tension, heart rate, and respiratory rate—all the things that seemed to go up when he was in pain. He liked seeing his output on the computer screen and learned how to evoke a relaxation response in his body, in part by breathing differently. The results were convincing because he could see how numbers changed, and he could connect that to how he felt—more relaxed! He began using the skills every day at home as his therapist suggested. He was pleased that his migraines were happening less often. Even better, his hip pain was less bothersome, and he was able to do a little more around the house during the day. He was even starting to get back to doing those rehab exercises his surgeon had told him to do months ago.

KEY POINTS

- Neuroimaging research shows that MBSR, mindfulness meditation, and hypnosis effectively alter pain processing activity.
- MBSR is highly structured and includes a range of therapeutic techniques, including mindfulness, movement components, and relaxation training.
- Although hypnosis is best studied for acute pain, some chronic pain research has suggested lasting effects.
- Biofeedback is a procedure that helps patients gain mastery over their ability to engage their healing and calming PNS through relaxation. Doing so counteracts the sympathetic nervous system and its negative effects on pain and stress.

■ Because biofeedback has a physiological emphasis, it may be better accepted by patients who otherwise resist psychological treatment approaches for pain.

RESOURCES

Mindfulness

MBSR and meditation resources:

Free online MBSR 8-week course: https://palousemindfulness.com/

Free mindfulness app:

MindApps. (2018). The Mindfulness App (Version 4.7.004) [Mobile application software]. Retrieved from https://www.apple.com/itunes

Free guided meditations (in English and Spanish), MBSR videos, and resources from the University of California, Los Angeles are available online (see http://marc.ucla.edu/mindful-meditations).

Headspace Guided Meditation (https://www.headspace.com/), available for purchase at https://www.apple.com/itunes.

Mindful.org offers a wealth of mindfulness information, videos, and tips on how to get started (see https://www.mindful.org/meditation/mindfulness-getting-started/).

Kabat-Zinn, J. (2013). *Full catastrophe living: Using the wisdom of your body and mind to face stress, pain, and illness.* New York, NY: Penguin Random House.

Hypnosis

Jensen, M. P., & Patterson, D. R. (2014). Hypnotic approaches for chronic pain management: Clinical implications of recent research findings. *American Psychologist, 69,* 167–177. Retrieved from http://www.apa.org/pubs/journals/releases/amp-a0035644.pdf

Spiegel, H., & Spiegel, D. (2004). *Trance and treatment: Clinical uses of hypnosis* (2nd ed.). Washington, DC: American Psychiatric Association Publishing.

Biofeedback

Locate a certified biofeedback therapist at http://www.bcia.org. Go to the "Find a Practitioner" tab and conduct a radius search based on the client's zip code.

Biofeedback for migraine. The American Migraine Foundation: https://americanmigrainefoundation.org/understanding-migraine/biofeedback-and-relaxation-training-for-headaches/

Sherman, R. A., & Hermann, C. (n.d.). *Clinical efficacy of psychophysiological assessments and biofeedback intervention for chronic pain disorders other than head area pain.* Retrieved from https://www.aapb.org/files/public/ReviewOfBFBForPain.pdf

8

Sleep and Fatigue

Up to 85% of people with chronic pain experience sleep problems (M. T. Smith & Haythornthwaite, 2004). Comorbid chronic pain and insomnia are associated with greater pain intensity, disability, anxiety, and depression. Sleep disturbance is an important therapeutic target because of its direct and indirect influence on chronic pain. Cognitive behavioral therapy for insomnia (CBTi) is an evidence-based psychobehavioral treatment for sleep that has been endorsed as the first-line treatment for chronic insomnia by National Institutes of Health consensus and the British Medical Association. Rooted in the science of behavior change, psychological theories, and the science of sleep, CBTi may be beneficial for patients with comorbid pain and sleep problems (Siebern & Manber, 2011). Helping patients disentangle the factors that contribute to poor sleep is a crucial to pain management. Simply put, better sleep means less pain. And poor sleep causes debilitating daytime fatigue. Often patients with chronic pain will note that fatigue—perhaps more

http://dx.doi.org/10.1037/0000104-009
Psychological Treatment for Patients With Chronic Pain, by B. D. Darnall

so than pain—prevents them from engaging in meaningful life activities and contributes to social withdrawal and isolation.

Sleep and pain are closely related. In fact, one of the best predictors of current pain intensity is the quality of sleep the night before. In turn, greater pain then leads to greater sleep disruption (Affleck, Urrows, Tennen, Higgins, & Abeles, 1996), in part due to "microarousals" that occur during sleep. Though the relationship between sleep and pain is bidirectional, the strongest association appears to be in the direction of poor sleep contributing to greater next-day pain, which can be counterintuitive for most patients. It is common for people to have a keen awareness of how pain affects their ability to fall and stay asleep. Less appreciated are the strong effects that poor sleep has on pain intensity and related factors. For instance, research has suggested that poor sleep is strongly associated with pain interference—and that this is accounted for by fatigue.

Once established, a self-sustaining cycle of poor sleep and greater pain may contribute to other problems. It is thought that poor sleep contributes to increased stress hormones, such as cortisol, and systemic inflammation, both of which negatively affect pain. Poor sleep contributes to anxiety and mood disorders and is a diagnostic criterion for both.

CIRCADIAN RHYTHM REGULATION FOR SLEEP, FATIGUE, AND PAIN

Increasingly, research findings point to the importance of regulating circadian rhythms for improving sleep and reducing fatigue (Segal, Tresidder, Bhatt, Gilron, & Ghasemlou, 2018). Pain-related sleep disturbance and various lifestyle choices can maintain and worsen circadian rhythm disruptions. Circadian rhythms can be disrupted by large changes in sleep patterns, such as jet lag, or from ongoing nightly sleep disruption from chronic pain. The over-the-counter supplement melatonin has been shown to help reset normal circadian rhythms necessary for good sleep and fatigue control (Jahanban-Esfahlan et al., 2017). Evidence suggests that exposure to bright light and early morning exercise may improve circadian regulation and facilitate nighttime sleep (Youngstedt et al., 2016).

Assessing sleep and related factors can reveal opportunities to improve both sleep and pain. Such factors include sleep hygiene practices, the environment, psychosocial and behavioral factors, and medications.

SLEEP APNEA IN CHRONIC PAIN

Poor sleep, difficulty awakening, and extreme daytime fatigue may be symptoms of underlying sleep central or obstructive sleep apnea. Some research suggests that between 50% and 80% of patients with chronic pain have obstructive sleep apnea (M. Roizenblatt, Rosa Neto, Tufik, & Roizenblatt, 2012; S. Roizenblatt, Rosa Neto, & Tufik, 2011). Left untreated, sleep apnea leads to lower oxygen intake throughout the night, greatly disrupted sleep cycles, poor sleep quality, greater daytime pain, and increased risk of other diseases. Being overweight increases the risk of obstructive sleep apnea. Patients can receive sleep evaluation at a sleep medicine clinic. If apnea is diagnosed, a sleep appliance may be prescribed (a continuous positive airway pressure device [CPAP] or bilevel positive airway pressure device). Prospective studies show that the use of sleep appliances reduces next-day pain.

OPIOIDS AND SLEEP DISRUPTION

Opioids are known to disrupt sleep architecture, thereby preventing patients from reaching the deeper stages of restorative sleep (Dimsdale, Norman, DeJardin, & Wallace, 2007; M. T. Smith & Quartana, 2010; Wang & Teichtahl, 2007; Webster, Choi, Desai, Webster, & Grant, 2008). Deep, restful sleep is needed to support overall health, good mood, energy, immune support, pain control, and physical and mental restoration. Patients may take opioids to reduce nighttime pain and facilitate sleep, yet the negative impact of opioids on sleep is insidious and can contribute to next-day fatigue and greater pain (Alattar & Scharf, 2009; Cheatle & Webster, 2015; Guilleminault, Cao, Yue, & Chawla, 2010; Mills et al., 2007; Mogri, Khan, Grant, & Mador, 2008; Wang & Teichtahl, 2007; Wang et al., 2005, 2008; Webster et al., 2008). For patients with sleep problems, nonopioid pain management strategies are recommended as first-line agents (Dowell, Haegerich, & Chou, 2016). It is also worth noting that opioids are not approved for prescription as sleep agents. Some research has suggested that with a slow, gentle opioid wean, sleep and pain control actually improve (Javaheri & Patel, 2017; Murphy, Clark, & Banou, 2013).

CLINICAL CHECKLIST
FOR SLEEP AND FATIGUE

- Assess sleep status and schedule. Ask patients about sleep habits and experience, including the number of hours slept each night and the regularity of their sleep schedule.
- Assess sleep quality and sleep disruption. Ask whether pain is contributing to interference with sleep onset or maintenance.
- Assess whether reactions to pain are compounding the problem (e.g., catastrophizing pain or dreading bedtime, muscle tension).
- Assess whether mental activity or anxiety is a contributing factor. Often, patients simply have a hard time quieting their mind at night, and this can be addressed with relaxation techniques.
- Assess caffeine consumption. Patients may rely on caffeine to combat fatigue. Caffeine can worsen pain and sleep problems, so use should be minimized. Rather, good sleep hygiene, good nutrition, hydration, daily relaxation response skills use, and graded activity are recommended to reduce fatigue.
- Assess for alcohol use. Alcohol use should be stopped during efforts to regulate circadian rhythms and good sleep cycles. Alcohol use at night erodes sleep quality and contributes to next-day fatigue.
- Assess whether the patient has had a sleep study and is adhering to medical recommendations, such as the use of a breathing appliance at bedtime (for apnea).
- Sedating medications may be a major contributor to fatigue. Encourage patients to discuss their fatigue with their prescribing physician and whether any medication changes can help (e.g., taking the

most sedating medications at bedtime or switching to less sedating medications).

GOOD SLEEP HYGIENE PRINCIPLES[1]

Many aspects of treatment for dysregulated sleep in chronic pain dovetail with general principles for good sleep hygiene, as follows:

- Adhere to a regular sleep schedule. Wake up at a fixed, early hour.
- Avoid daytime naps.
- Daytime movement and exercise is beneficial for sleep and reduces fatigue.
- A cool, quiet environment is best for sleep. Custom silicone earplugs may benefit those who are sensitive to noise.
- Finish dinner at least 2 hours before bedtime.
- No caffeine for 8 to 10 hours before bedtime.
- Avoid alcohol. A byproduct of alcohol metabolism is a stimulant that serves to disrupt sleep.
- Avoid bright light and blue light exposure in the evening. No computers or smartphones 1 hour before bed.
- Make nighttime relaxing: Try meditation, a warm bath, reading, or other relaxation activities that prepare mind and body for sleep.
- Practice deep (diaphragmatic) breathing at bedtime.
- Save difficult conversations and stimulating TV or movies for daytime or early evening only.
- Stop use of electronic devices (e.g., smartphones, iPads, computers) at least 1 hour before bedtime.
- The bed should be used for sleep and intercourse only (not for TV watching, work, or smartphone use).
- If sleep onset is delayed, encourage patients to leave the bed for another room to do light reading or any boring activity until ready for sleep.

---

[1]From *The Opioid-Free Pain Relief Kit: 10 Simple Steps to Ease Your Pain* (pp. 60–62), by B. Darnall, 2016, Boulder, CO: Bull Publishing Company. Copyright 2016 by Bull Publishing Company. Adapted with permission.

- Sleep balance is key. Too much sleep is as problematic as getting too little. Hypersomnia can be a sign of major depression, overmedication, or an underlying medical condition. Although medical evaluation is encouraged, the psychological evaluation may assess for mood, medication use, and other behavioral factors.

Consider referring patients for CBTi for in-depth psychobehavioral treatment for sleep. CBTi is first-line evidence-based treatment for insomnia. Finally, you may consider recommending the patient obtain a medical sleep study to rule out any sleep problems that may require medical attention.

KEY POINTS

- Sleep disorders contribute to greater pain, fatigue, and poor mood. Assessing and treating sleep dysfunction is an essential component of pain management and self-management of pain. Where possible, address sleep issues first.
- Optimize sleep hygiene.
- Pain is often worse later in the day and particularly at bedtime because of the lack of distractions and sometimes fatigue.
- Assess and address psychological factors that may be contributing to poor sleep, such as catastrophizing nighttime pain and dreading sleep time.
- Evoking the relaxation response at bedtime can help reduce the psychological and physiological factors that amplify pain and insomnia.
- Sleep apnea is common in chronic pain. Risk factors include being overweight and using opioids.
- Encourage an evaluation with a sleep physician for patients with poor sleep and extreme daytime fatigue.
- For patients who have been prescribed a sleep appliance (e.g., CPAP), encourage the use of the device as a pathway to reduce daytime pain.
- Alcohol and opioids disrupt sleep architecture, thereby impeding the restorative stages of sleep. Opioid cessation has been shown to reverse sleep apnea.

■ Restoring normal circadian rhythms with good sleep hygiene principles, early morning exercise and bright light exposure, and nighttime melatonin use may improve sleep and fatigue and reduce pain.

RESOURCES

Patient workbook:

Carney, C., & Manber, R. (2009). *Quiet your mind and get to sleep: Solutions to insomnia for those with depression, anxiety or chronic pain.* Oakland, CA: New Harbinger.

Free CBT sleep app that provides sleep education and guides users to develop positive habits that improve sleep:

U.S. Department of Veterans Affairs. (2018). CBT-i Coach (Version 2.3) [Mobile application software]. Retrieved from https://www.apple.com/itunes

9

Opioids

*O*pioids are medications that reduce pain and affect reward pathways in the brain. Opioids are most effective for short-term pain relief (see Table 2.2 for a list of generic and brand name opioid drugs). Long-term opioid use can be highly problematic because it is associated with a host of health risks, some of which contribute to worsening pain. As noted in Chapter 2, opioids can contribute to medical complexity and *polypharmacy*—wherein more and more medications are prescribed to treat the side effects of previous medications (see Figure 2.1).

HEALTH RISKS ASSOCIATED WITH LONG-TERM OPIOID USE

Although most people are aware of the risks for opioid addiction, few patients and even few health care providers are aware of the broader array

http://dx.doi.org/10.1037/0000104-010
Psychological Treatment for Patients With Chronic Pain, by B. D. Darnall

of health risks associated with long-term opioid use for chronic pain. These risks include

- hormone disruption,
- sleep disturbance and sleep apnea,
- depression (new-onset depression or recurrence of depression),
- anxiety,
- greater pain sensitivity,
- addiction,
- tolerance and dependence,
- slowed cognitive functioning,
- narcotic bowel syndrome and severe constipation, and
- unintentional overdose and overdose death.

Opioids have direct and indirect psychological effects. For instance, opioids cause hormonal dysregulation and sleep disturbance, and indirectly these can affect mood, anxiety, and behavior.

OPIOID RESTRICTIONS

Opioids are scheduled drugs that require Drug Enforcement Agency (DEA) and Food and Drug Administration oversight and require physicians to have special prescribing licenses. These rules were established because prescription opioids are abused by those seeking to achieve a "high." As such, prescription opioids have great street value when sold illegally. State and federal guidelines exist regarding dose limits for opioid prescriptions for chronic pain. In recent years, opioid overprescribing—too many prescriptions and at risky doses—contributed to a fraction of patients becoming addicted and to unintentional overdose deaths, often from patients unwittingly combining prescribed medications (even taken

Research has shown that, on average, opioids reduce pain by only about 25%—about the same as psychobehavioral treatment, yet opioids carry substantial health risks.

exactly as prescribed, opioids combined with other drugs can be a deadly combination; Sun et al., 2017).

OPIOID AGREEMENTS

Prescribing physicians often require patients to sign an "opioid agreement" before prescribing opioids. An opioid agreement includes parameters designating how the medications will be prescribed and used and expectations regarding patient behavior. For instance, prescribers often require regular urine drug tests. Urine drug tests tell prescribers two things: (a) whether opioids are in the patient's system as they should be—if not, there may be reason to suspect that the medication is being diverted for sale; and (b) whether illicit drugs are being taken in combination with opioids. For example, a "positive" result for cocaine would stand in direct violation of the signed opioid agreement. Of course, the vast majority of patients with chronic pain are neither diverting nor taking illicit drugs—they are taking their medications exactly as prescribed and adhering to their opioid agreement. As such, patients may experience drug testing as insulting and humiliating.

Opioids are commonly referred to as *painkillers*, but this term is a misnomer. Rarely is pain eliminated with opioids. Up to 30% of people who try opioids are unable to tolerate the side effects and stop them fairly quickly. Even when side effects are tolerated or low, research has shown that, on average, opioids reduce pain only by about 25% to 30% (Kalso, Edwards, Moore, & McQuay, 2004)—about the same as reported by some studies on cognitive behavioral therapy. The term *painkiller* also perpetuates false beliefs that medications are the total solution and that persistent pain indicates a need for higher doses. In fact, higher opioid doses offer most patients with chronic pain little more than greater health risks.

Patients with mental health diagnoses, such as major depression, anxiety, and posttraumatic stress disorder, are between 2 and 8 times more likely to be prescribed opioids for chronic pain than patients without mental health diagnoses (Braden et al., 2008; Breckenridge & Clark, 2003; M. D. Sullivan et al., 2008). Patients with comorbid chronic pain, mental health conditions, and prescribed opioids are at greater risk of prolonged opioid use, opioid misuse, and addiction (Edlund, Martin, Fan, Braden, et al., 2010; M. D. Sullivan et al., 2010). Because emotional pain and physical pain are experienced similarly (and are bidirectionally related), patients have increased risk of unwittingly taking prescribed opioids to medicate emotional distress that is related to their pain.

OPIOID PHYSICAL DEPENDENCE AND TOLERANCE

Physical dependence and tolerance are commonly experienced by patients taking long-term opioids and are not an indication of addiction. Physical dependence on opioids occurs as the body becomes accustomed to having stable doses of opioids, and when the opioid dose is lowered abruptly, withdrawal symptoms occur (e.g., anxiety, greater pain, agitation, nausea, chills, rapid heart rate, inability to sleep). Patients may worry that experiencing opioid withdrawal symptoms after missing a medication dose provides evidence that they are addicted to opioids. Not true. Withdrawal symptoms are neither "proof" that one is addicted nor is it a sign that one cannot get off opioids. Care must be taken to reduce opioids sensibly, maximize patient physical and psychological comfort, and obviate the experience of withdrawal symptoms.

Tolerance occurs as the body becomes accustomed to opioids and larger doses are needed to achieve the same amount of pain relief. Opioids may cause greater pain sensitivity, and this can lead to risky dose escalation. If opioids are not providing sufficient pain relief at low doses, often a better and safer strategy is to focus on nonopioid pain treatments.

A slippery slope: Even though relief is felt when a single dose of opioids is taken, long-term use often leads to tolerance (i.e., needing more of the medication over time) and for some people, worsening pain. Both lead to risky opioid dose escalation in an attempt to gain relief.

OPIOID USE DISORDER AND ADDICTION

Physical dependence and opioid tolerance are distinct from addiction and opioid use disorder (see the fifth edition of the *Diagnostic and Statistical Manual of Mental Disorders* [American Psychiatric Association, 2013]). To confirm an addiction or opioid use disorder diagnosis, additional symptoms and behaviors must be involved, such as violating opioid contracts, "losing" prescriptions, exceeding prescribed doses, doctor shopping, using illicit substances, and buying opioids illegally. Common myths about prescription opioid addiction risks are described and debunked in Exhibit 9.1.

OPIOID STIGMA

Opioids are a source of medical and social stigma, and patients may find themselves feeling marginalized by others' judgments about opioids. Some patients describe feeling that they are treated like addicts for taking prescribed opioids, sometimes within the medical system itself. Addressing feelings of injustice, anger, or shame related to opioid use may be important

---

Exhibit 9.1

Opioid Myths and Truths

Myth: Pain protects patients from addiction to their opioid medications.

Truth: Addiction to opioids can occur even when they are taken as prescribed.

Myth: Only long-term use of certain opioids leads to addiction.

Truth: All opioids carry risk for addiction.

Myth: Only patients with certain characteristics are vulnerable to addiction.

Truth: Though some patients are more vulnerable, no patient is immune to opioid addiction.

Note. From "Opioid Abuse in Chronic Pain—Misconceptions and Mitigation Strategies," by N. D. Volkow and A. T. McLellan, 2016, *New England Journal of Medicine, 374,* p. 1254. Copyright 2016 by the Massachusetts Medical Society. Adapted with permission.

therapeutic topics. In 2016, the Centers for Disease Control and Prevention, the DEA, and state agencies established guidelines and prescribing limits on opioids. The guidelines cited a lack of data showing a lack of benefit associated with long-term opioid use: On average, pain was not improving, function was not improving, and patient risks were skyrocketing. Consequently, patients who had been prescribed opioids for years or even decades were suddenly told that their established pain care plan was no longer acceptable and must be abruptly changed. Anger and fear are common emotional responses to treatments being taken away, particularly when patients say they work for them, despite the research data. Fear about tapering prescription opioids—or having them taken away—is the most common medication concern reported by patients who take opioids.

PATIENTS' FEARS ABOUT REDUCING OPIOIDS

Patients taking opioids may have great fear about reducing opioids or having them "taken away." A common belief is that reducing opioids will leave them with uncontrolled pain. In many cases, this message is learned through experience. They may have tried to stop opioids on their own— often cold turkey or too fast—and went into withdrawal. The main withdrawal symptom is greater pain. However, people often mistakenly believe this temporary increased pain due to withdrawal is their "baseline pain level" without opioids. This misunderstanding can serve to increase pain and anxiety and perpetuates a false belief that fewer opioids mean worse pain. In fact, the data show that when opioids are reduced slowly, sensibly, and supportively, pain either stays the same or decreases—even for patients who have taken high dose opioids for years (Darnall et al., 2018; Murphy, Clark, & Banou, 2013).

Typically, patients taking or considering taking opioids lack education about opioid risks and consequences and therefore are not making informed choices. I have treated numerous patients who, after taking opioids for years, were indignant that opioids had worsened existing problems and created new ones for them. However, some patients who have been appropriately prescribed opioids have found that any tradeoffs were worth the benefit they gained. There are no absolutes with opioid therapy for chronic pain. Although they should be avoided in general, opioids can have a role for carefully selected patients with chronic pain. Three important factors should be considered:

- Even if opioids are appropriate therapy, patients should be given full information about risks and consequences of opioids so they can make informed choices. I wrote *Less Pain, Fewer Pills* (Darnall, 2014a) specifically for patients considering opioids and for those taking opioids who wish to reduce their use of them by optimizing psychobehavioral strategies.

- Assess the benefits. Opioids should help patients function better, or it is unlikely that the risks are worth the benefit. Recognizing that you are not the prescriber, evaluating for functional improvements can help you discuss this issue more with your client and, when relevant and appropriate, their physician.

- Psychobehavioral strategies, physical therapies, and self-management should be optimized to minimize need for and use of the medications and, therefore, patient risks (Darnall, 2014b). Anxiety and behavioral pain management strategies should be implemented in patients taking opioids who wish to taper down or stop them. For opioid tapering to be successful, patient fears and concerns should be addressed (Darnall et al., 2018). Effective strategies include reducing opioid doses very slowly and emphasizing daily use of psychobehavioral skills to self-manage symptoms and distress. Unless there is medical urgency, slow opioid tapering that stretches over 6 months or more can allow patients adequate time to adjust biologically and psychologically. A slow taper schedule and ongoing psychological support are crucial for patients who may have underlying anxiety, posttraumatic stress disorder, or other psychobehavioral factors that may be unmasked as opioids are reduced.

Cautionary notes for therapists include the need to evaluate patients taking opioids for concomitant medications and behaviors that could be problematic or fatal.

CLINICAL CHECKLIST

- **Assess for chronic pain and opioid use.** Ask clients whether they have ongoing pain. If so, ask what their current treatment regimen is and whether they are prescribed opioids.
- **Evaluate for alcohol use.** Opioids and alcohol are both central nervous system depressants. Alcohol should never be used while taking opioids because respiratory arrest and death can occur during sleep. Provide education to patients and communicate with prescribers, if appropriate.
- **Evaluate for concurrent use of benzodiazepines.** Concurrent use of prescription opioids and benzodiazepines is the most common cause of overdose and death from prescription opioids (Sun et al., 2017). Benzodiazepines are most commonly prescribed to treat anxiety, even though long-term use for anxiety is discouraged. Like opioids, benzodiazepines are central nervous system depressants. Research has shown that when taken together, the risks of respiratory depression are exponential because they have synergistic effects that increase the effects of both and make unintentional overdose easy. Unintentional overdose risks are higher in patients who are forgetful or knowingly take an additional dose of either medication. Combining opioids and benzodiazepines can be fatal even in low doses. Anxiety is common in patients with chronic pain, thereby underscoring the need to evaluate anxiolytic medications and optimize behavioral treatment for anxiety and pain. Alert patients that there are health risks with taking these two medications, and encourage them to discuss this with their doctor or prescriber or assess their willingness to allow you to discuss with their prescriber. To reduce risks, best practice is to consider weaning off one of the medications—slowly—while under medical supervision and close psychological care. See Table 9.1 for a list of generic and brand-name benzodiazepines.
- **Evaluate for substance use disorder and opioid use disorder.** Red flag symptoms include taking more medication than is prescribed, doctor shopping, breaking opioid contracts, "losing" opioid prescriptions, visiting emergency rooms for more opioids, alcohol use, use of illicit drugs, and obtaining opioids illegally. Unless you treat addiction,

Table 9.1
Benzodiazepine Medications

Generic benzodiazepines	Benzodiazepine drug brand name
Alprazolam	Xanax
Clonazepam	Klonopin
Diazepam	Valium
Lorazepam	Ativan
Temazepam	Restoril

psychotherapy is unlikely to be productive in the presence of an active substance use disorder. Consider referral to an addictionologist or addiction psychologist.

- **Evaluate for psychological disorders and behaviors.** Evaluation for psychological disorders is particularly relevant in cases in which you may be asked to determine whether a patient is an appropriate candidate for initiation of an opioid prescription. Or clients may mention that they have spoken with their doctor and are considering starting opioids to treat their chronic pain. Strong overlap exists between pain, opioid prescription and dose, and psychological disorders. As such, new opioid prescriptions are contraindicated in patients with a history of substance use disorder and opioid use disorder. At minimum, encourage your patients to discuss these risks with their doctor. In select cases, and only when appropriate permissions are in place, you may consider discussing with the patient's physician.
- **Help your patients reduce their health risks by encouraging a psychobehavioral approach to pain management.** Ideally, evidence-based psychobehavioral treatment for pain is the first line of treatment, before opioids are started. However, even if opioids were prescribed years ago, evidence-based psychological approaches can help patients reduce their need and use of opioids.
- **There are special risks for surgery in clients with a history of substance use disorder.** For clients with a history of substance use disorder, close

monitoring must be exercised in cases in which opioids are unavoidable, such as after major surgery. Discuss with clients how their psychological history creates a risk of prolonged opioid use after surgery and possibly addiction recurrence. When indicated and appropriate permissions are in place, consider establishing care coordination with other members of the patient's health care team before surgery. Everyone shares the same goal of helping the patient achieve best surgical outcomes with the lowest risks. Recommend working with the patient to optimize behavioral strategies (or referring as needed to a specialist) and increasing the frequency of therapy visits until opioids are stopped.

SUSAN'S STORY

Susan was a 46-year-old high-powered attorney who had stopped practicing law to stay home and raise her three children.[1] She had chronic pain from several medical conditions, including degeneration in her cervical spine (neck) and fibromyalgia. Staying at home seemed like a practical decision for the entire household, and as her pain increased, she was glad she was not working long hours at the office.

Susan was in distress when I met her. She felt out of control and anxious and was taking Xanax for anxiety and Ambien for insomnia. She was also taking high doses of opioids for her neck and shoulder pain as well as using a fentanyl Duragesic patch that delivers opioids through the skin. She was in a vicious cycle: Her anxiety was making her pain worse, and her pain was making her more anxious. Despite all the medication she was taking, her pain was still severe, as was her stress level at home.

"I need to gain control over my pain and my life, but I have no idea how to do this," she said. "I feel like I'm doing everything, yet nothing is working." She was either pushing herself to do things in spite of her pain, or she was in bed trying to recover from a pain flare brought on by having pushed herself so hard. In either case, she was struggling, and her constant struggle was sucking the joy out of her life.

---

[1]The case example used in this chapter is fictitious or has been disguised to protect confidentiality. It is derived from an account first published in *Less Pain, Fewer Pills: Avoid the Dangers of Prescription Opioids and Gain Control Over Chronic Pain*, by B. Darnall, 2014a, pp. 86–92. Copyright 2014 by Bull Publishing Company. Reprinted with permission.

Susan's pain and suffering were particularly distressing to her because she had always been in control of her life—until now. Her doctor was unhappy with all the medication she was taking, and she was viewed as a classic "problem pain patient." She had an alert placed in her medical chart to warn her medical providers that she was on a special opioid agreement—a clear indicator of a patient who was "noncompliant" with her opioids. She wanted her life back and herself back, but she could not imagine getting off the opioids with such constant and severe pain.

Susan attended a single-session pain class I gave at her primary care doctor's office. In the class, she learned how she was participating in her pain. She learned that, in big and small ways, she had more influence over her pain than she realized. She found she could change her pain—for better or for worse—by changing her emotions, her thoughts, and her choices. Susan contacted me after the class and asked to meet individually. I met with her for private sessions every 2 weeks for several months.

The Body

In the first session Susan learned that—like most people with chronic pain—the way she was responding to her pain and her stress was automatic and unhelpful. She learned how to control her reactions and, in doing so, gained control over her experience. After years of being prescribed medications to change her levels of physical and emotional distress, Susan was surprised to learn she could calm her mind and her body without a pill (you too will learn how to do this). I gave her a pain management audio CD and asked her to listen to it at least once daily and ideally more often than that because she had so much anxiety. By listening to the CD regularly, she was retraining her mind and body with methods proven to reduce pain and suffering. A big contributor to Susan's neck pain was the load of tension she carried in her neck muscles. Regular use of the audio CD allowed her to begin releasing her neck tension, thus reducing her pain. She learned to turn her awareness into her body and to detect what her body needed so that she could begin taking better care of it.

The Day-to-Day

Next, we focused on what was happening in her daily life. Susan acknowledged that she did a lot for her family—too much, in fact. Her children did few, if any, chores. Susan was the household cook, chauffeur, and maid, despite the fact that her kids were fully able-bodied and ages 13, 16, and 17. She had trained her children to expect her to do all the work for them. She was enmeshed with her kids and was unable to maintain good boundaries with them. She would cave in when faced with their disappointment or disapproval. She was bewildered at how she could stop the cycle. "I've asked them to do more around the house, but it never happens," she lamented. Instead, she would fall back into her role as servant. This was the first thing we aimed to change.

I coached Susan to stop picking up the slack for others, literally and figuratively. She began leaving their dirty laundry piled up in their bedrooms. If they needed clean clothes, they were forced to do the wash themselves. She stopped straightening up their rooms and instead began closing their doors so their messes did not encroach on her clean home. She stopped catering to her 16-year-old daughter's every whim—including driving her to school; she lovingly yet firmly informed her that she was to begin taking the bus. In doing so, Susan found she had time freed up for self-care, such as yoga and gym exercise. She began creating independence for herself while simultaneously encouraging greater independence for her kids.

This was a win–win for everyone. Her kids complained, but they had to begin taking on appropriate levels of responsibility. Susan found her family could tolerate being inconvenienced and that she could tolerate their disappointment. She stopped spending all her time and energy inappropriately catering to others. Setting firm limits with her children allowed her stress and her pain to lessen, for four reasons:

- She learned to set appropriate limits and was no longer pushing her body so hard in an effort to please her family and reduce her guilt. In doing so, she eliminated all the overwork that was pushing her into greater pain levels, and she also freed up time for herself.
- She took better care of herself and thus began meeting her own physical and emotional needs.

- She used the relaxation response audio CD twice daily and, in doing so, she reduced her anxiety, stress, and muscle tension and was falling asleep faster.
- As she reclaimed control over her life, she became calmer and more relaxed, and from this calm state, she made better decisions. Her choices supported better pain control, and she developed confidence in her ability to manage her pain, her emotions, and her stress. Her newfound confidence allowed her to become centered and grounded within herself.

Susan's progress with pain management meant she was able to meet her goal of tapering off her medications. She stopped the Xanax first. This was the easiest. As she managed her anxiety with the steps just outlined, her need for Xanax melted away. As her pain was better managed, she began cutting down on her fentanyl Duragesic patch—literally. Each time she placed a new patch, she took scissors and cut the patch smaller and smaller before applying it.[2] On her own and without her doctor's knowledge, she was tapering her dosing of fentanyl by cutting her patch a bit smaller each time (though this is not recommended). She acknowledged it was not easy, but she was determined to do it, and she was determined to change her life choices to make it possible.

Along the way, Susan realized how much her stress levels were linked to her opioid use. She noticed that when her daughter was being obstinate and argumentative, she would reach back to rub the fentanyl patch on her shoulder. "I know now that I was instinctively trying to medicate the stress by rubbing the patch to release more medication," she said.

The Mind

Susan learned how to change her thought patterns so that she was no longer catastrophizing her pain. Before I first met Susan, she worried about her pain getting worse, and she felt there was nothing she could do about it. She was not coping well mentally or emotionally, and her distress was

---

[2]A note to underscore that Susan's approach was not medically advised and is not recommended.

contributing to her pain and medication use. Through treatment, she learned how to keep her mind calm and how to help herself make choices that supported her primary goal: managing her stress and pain rather than catering to others. She also learned that by taking excellent care of herself, she was a great role model for her children. Before, her children were learning that it was OK for Mom to sacrifice herself—after all, she did not count or deserve to be taken care of. Now, they were learning that Mom deserved to be respected and well cared for. She was teaching them by example that excellent self-care is healthy and essential. Through her actions, she was modeling important, positive values that would shape their lives.

The Self

As Susan tapered off opioids, she began "feeling" more. She was surprised to feel joy at times and anger at times—healthy emotions! She acknowledged that the opioids had left her feeling somewhat numb—to physical sensation and also to her emotions. She was pleased to reconnect to a full spectrum of emotions.

Her anger turned out to be good information. It informed her that something in her life had to be addressed. So she began addressing things directly and appropriately and thus started nipping her stress in the bud. She developed a healthy level of assertiveness with her husband and kids, and although there were some growing pains, the whole family benefited. It is not healthy for anyone when a family member becomes numb and passive. As Susan began feeling more, she connected with her authentic self and started to realize what was missing in her life. She discovered she wanted to do more outside the home in a structured way, and now that her pain was better managed, she felt ready to realize this goal.

When I last saw Susan for follow-up, she reported that her blood pressure was much lower, to the point that her cardiologist was impressed and asked what her secret was. She was excited to tell me the secret was the work we did together. "It's really the result of all this work we've been doing in session and that I've been implementing at home—making life changes to reduce my stress and pain and to get off the prescriptions. I can't believe I have my life back," she told me.

One of the best things to come from all of Susan's progress was her surge in energy. She found she had more energy available to channel in productive ways, whether it was exercising, connecting with friends and family, doing the craftwork she loved, volunteering, or going back to work. "I was really surprised at how much energy the opioids robbed from me," she said.

Susan is inspiring. She still has her medical conditions and limitations, but she is living her best possible life. She tapered off her Xanax and Duragesic fentanyl and is now tapering off her Ambien. Instead of popping a pill to sleep, she is focusing on calming herself in the evening by turning off the TV and computer in the hour before bedtime. She is eating dinner earlier so she is not overly full at bedtime. She is listening to her relaxation audio CD before bed so that she readies her mind and her body for sleep. She is focusing on her making these changes herself so that she does not need to rely on the Ambien. Taking pills may seem easier on the surface, but Susan preferred to have her life back. And she preferred to know that she, not a medication, was in control of it. An important part of Susan's story was the fact that the stresses in her family caused her both emotional and physical pain. Only by addressing the emotional stress and social pain did she gain control over her physical pain and reduce her use of medications. Figure 9.1 shows the stress–pain–medication use cycle Susan's treatment had to address.

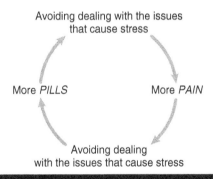

Figure 9.1

Stress and pain medication use. Susan's treatment involved breaking her stress–pain–medication use cycle. From *Less Pain, Fewer Pills: Avoid the Dangers of Prescription Opioids and Gain Control Over Chronic Pain* (p. 94), by B. Darnall, 2014, Boulder, CO: Bull Publishing Company. Copyright 2014 by Bull Publishing Company. Reprinted with permission.

KEY POINTS

- On average, opioids are of limited value for chronic pain.
- For select people, opioids are one component of an effective, comprehensive pain care plan.
- People with mental health diagnoses are more likely to be prescribed opioids and at risky doses.
- Multiple health risks (including addiction) exist for all people prescribed opioids.
- The following may reduce opioid risks: (a) optimizing psychobehavioral and nonpharmacologic pain management strategies; (b) avoiding beginning an opioid prescription where possible; (c) if prescribed, minimizing the use of opioids; (d) keeping doses low; (e) eliminating coprescription with benzodiazepines; (f) if opioids are not working, stopping them rather than escalating the dose; and (g) optimizing nonopioid medical strategies (e.g., nonopioid medication or interventions).
- Patient education about opioid risks and how to minimize them is critical. Recommend online and print resources to your patients so they may learn more and become empowered.

RESOURCES

Darnall, B. (2014). *Less pain, fewer pills: Avoid the dangers of prescription opioids and gain control over chronic pain*. Boulder, CO: Bull Publishing Company.

Darnall, B. (2016). *The opioid-free pain relief kit: 10 simple steps to ease your pain*. Boulder, CO: Bull Publishing Company.

Volkow, N. D., & McLellan, A. T. (2016). Opioid abuse in chronic pain—Misconceptions and mitigation strategies. *New England Journal of Medicine, 374*, 1253–1263. Retrieved from http://www.nejm.org/doi/pdf/10.1056/NEJMra1507771

10

Special Populations, Substance Use, and Substance Use Disorder

This chapter discusses some additional considerations for special populations that constitute a substantial fraction of the total chronic pain population. Older adults, minorities, and individuals with current substance use or current or historical substance use disorder (SUD) merit specific assessment and treatment considerations.

SPECIAL POPULATIONS

Older Adults

International studies have revealed that up to 75% of adults 65 years and older report living with persistent pain (Tsang et al., 2008). The majority describe their pain as moderate, and about a quarter report having severe pain. Older adults are more likely to have additional health problems that can cause or complicate chronic pain and associated polypharmacy

http://dx.doi.org/10.1037/0000104-011
Psychological Treatment for Patients With Chronic Pain, by B. D. Darnall
Copyright © 2019 by the American Psychological Association. All rights reserved.

(Held et al., 2017; Kim & Parish, 2017). When cognitive impairment is a concern, assessment should include potential polypharmacy, the impact of pain, and depression ("pseudodementia") because each factor may independently negatively affect memory and other cognitive faculties.

Older adults are also more likely to have frailty, mobility, and balance issues, and each may affect their ability to engage in daily therapeutic exercise and other self-care activities (Tannenbaum, 2013). Behavioral pain treatment principles are highly relevant in older adults because of the greater prevalence and severity of pain. Older adults may be more likely to have a stoic attitude about pain and attribute pain to "normal aging" and therefore avoid seeking treatment. Because many older adults minimize their experience of pain, it is important to assess for pain and to encourage treatment to improve quality of life, health, sleep, mood, and function.

Older adults may be resistant to pain medications and, like many people, be unaware that a multitude of other pain treatments exists, including nonpharmacologic treatments. Helping older adults engage in appropriate movement and exercise can be an important part of their pain and health management plan. Chronic pain self-management programs have been found to be effective in older adults (Nicholas et al., 2017). Individuals who are resistant to psychological treatment for pain may be more willing to try chronic pain self-management, in part because it is viewed as nonpsychological, and the groups tend to be led by (and composed of) older adult peers with chronic pain. An additional option is a free chronic pain support group, such as the peer-led American Chronic Pain Association support groups. Group treatments and supports can serve a dual purpose of enhancing social engagement in older adults who are isolated.

Racial and Ethnic Disparities

Racial and ethnic disparities in pain reporting and pain treatment have been well demonstrated (Campbell & Edwards, 2012; Green et al., 2003; Nguyen, Ugarte, Fuller, Haas, & Portenoy, 2005). On average, African Americans report greater pain sensitivity compared with Whites. Further, they are less likely to have their pain treated. Research has shown that pain in Whites is treated more aggressively than in non-Whites. In part, treatment disparities exist because of explicit or implicit medical provider bias. Minorities are more likely to have poorer overall health and related conditions that worsen pain, such as major depression. The literature suggests that lower socioeconomic status may account for many racial disparities in pain and health (Institute of Medicine [US] Committee on Advancing Pain Research, Care, and Education, 2011). Pain is more likely to be disabling in those with low incomes or less than high school education. Finally, compared to Caucasians, African Americans were 3 times more likely to report racism as being a major problem in health care (and Hispanics were twice as likely), and distrust of the medical system may discourage minorities from seeking medical care in the first place (LaVeist, Nickerson, & Bowie, 2000).

SUBSTANCE USE AND SUBSTANCE USE DISORDER

Alcohol

Individuals with chronic pain may report using alcohol or illicit substances to manage their pain. Using alcohol to manage pain has been shown to contribute to alcohol use problems (Brennan, Schutte, & Moos, 2005). Studies show that prolonged use of alcohol and drug use has been associated with greater pain intensity (Morasco, Turk, Donovan, & Dobscha, 2013). Alcohol use can also contribute to poor sleep and next-day fatigue (Miller et al., 2017; Thakkar, Sharma, & Sahota, 2015). Moreover, alcohol use is contraindicated with most pharmaceuticals, in particular, opioids, benzodiazepines, and other central nervous system depressant agents.

Medical Marijuana and Cannabis

The decriminalization of marijuana has led to an increase in its use for pain control, and efforts to minimize opioid prescribing have likely played a role, as well. Findings from one study suggested that 15% of Canadians with chronic pain and 30% of British patients with multiple sclerosis reported medical marijuana use (Park & Wu, 2017). Even though state laws may allow the recreational and medical use of marijuana, standing federal criminal laws prevent many physicians from endorsing cannabis for their patients. Perhaps more important, other factors prevent many physicians from sanctioning cannabis use. First, rigid federal laws have impeded large clinical trials, and therefore the science on safety, efficacy, and dosing is lacking. Second, because cannabis is not regulated like a pharmaceutical, there are no standards for licensing, safety, potency, and dosing. Prescribers cannot assure patients safe and accurate dosing because no such system exists.

Despite the lack of systems and regulations, some patients report substantial pain relief with cannabis use. Marijuana is a psychoactive drug and therefore should be avoided in individuals with current or past SUD. Caution is noted for patients taking long-term opioids: Medical marijuana use has been associated with prescription opioid misuse (Nugent et al., 2018). Marijuana or cannabis derivatives that have psychoactive compounds (THC) removed are preferred. Psychologists should assess for improved pain, mood, and function and reflect observations to patients with pain who may be using cannabis derivatives.

Some cautions for analgesic cannabis use are as follows:

- Cigarette smoking is associated with greater pain and poorer outcomes (Hooten et al., 2009; Weingarten et al., 2008). Patients who smoke cigarettes or marijuana should be given education and encouraged to stop smoking as a pathway for pain relief. Smoking should never be part of a pain care plan.
- Medical marijuana use may contribute to apathy, fatigue, depression, and disability in some individuals, particularly with heavy use. Assess the level of marijuana use, engagement in daily activities, and SUD.

SUBSTANCE USE DISORDER

All patients with chronic pain should be assessed for current SUD as well as history of SUD. A national study of more than 1,400 patients seeking treatment for opioid use disorder found that 60% reported that their first exposure to opioids was a medical prescription for legitimate pain (Cicero, Lynskey, Todorov, Inciardi, & Surratt, 2008).

Studies have suggested that between 20% and 30% of patients with chronic pain have a current SUD. The rate increases to 40% to 50% when considering patients with chronic pain who have a history of SUD. A history of SUD also confers risk of poorer pain outcomes and greater treatment needs (Morasco et al., 2013, 2017). SUDs commonly occur with other mental health disorders, such as depression or posttraumatic stress disorder, with dual diagnoses requiring additional treatments. Recently there has been more focus on identifying and treating patients with "triple diagnoses": chronic pain, SUD, and other psychopathology. Studies have suggested that individuals with chronic pain and comorbid SUD require more intensive treatment for their function to improve. In treatment, the underlying psychobehavioral factors that are serving to amplify pain and SUD are addressed. Patients with SUD may be suitable for group psychological treatment for pain once the patient is committed to abstinence and their behavior is stable.

See Chapter 10 for additional detail on opioids and SUD. Opioids are contraindicated in individuals with SUD and avoided whenever possible (Morasco et al., 2013). For cases in which opioids cannot be avoided (e.g., after major surgery), the patient's physician should be aware of the SUD and (ideally) closely monitor the administration of a minimal amount of pills. Frequent psychological follow-up and support meetings (such as Alcoholics Anonymous) may help prevent relapse or worsening of SUD due to exposure to prescription opioids. Assess for the use of substances and opioids at each follow-up.

KEY POINTS

- Up to 75% of older adults have ongoing pain.
- Race, lower socioeconomic status, and lower levels of education are associated with greater pain.
- Older adults and racial minorities are less likely to report their pain and thus may be suffering silently.
- Special populations may be less aware of psychobehavioral treatment for chronic pain; be sure to provide education about psychobehavioral treatment options.

- Racial bias (implicit and explicit) in medical care has fostered distrust among many minority individuals, and this may affect their willingness to seek care. For instance, research has suggested that pain is treated less aggressively for non-Whites than for Whites. Validating the patient experience and helping connect patients to pain care may be important aspects of therapy.
- Smoking and alcohol use are associated with greater pain; research has suggested that cessation of both may reduce pain and response to medical treatments.
- All patients with chronic pain should be assessed for substance use and SUD.
- Particularly in at-risk patients, assess current substance use at each follow-up.
- Even a history of SUD is associated with poorer outcomes and requires a higher level of care.
- SUD and chronic pain are mutually maintaining. SUD worsens pain, and pain triggers cravings.
- Special risks exist for SUD relapse in patients with a history of SUD who are prescribed opioids after surgery. Opioid use should be minimized and closely monitored by prescribers and mental health professionals.

RESOURCES

Older Adults

Molton, I. R., & Terrill, A. L. (2014). Overview of persistent pain in older adults. *American Psychologist, 69,* 197–207. Retrieved from http://www.apa.org/pubs/journals/releases/amp-a0035794.pdf

Racial and Ethnic Disparities

Tait, R. C., & Chibnall, J. T. (2014). Racial/ethnic disparities in the assessment and treatment of pain: Psychosocial perspectives. *American Psychologist, 69,* 131–141. Retrieved from http://www.apa.org/pubs/journals/releases/amp-a0035204.pdf

Substance Use Disorders

Substance Abuse and Mental Health Services Administration. (2012). *Managing chronic pain in adults with or in recovery from substance use disorders.* Retrieved from https://store.samhsa.gov/shin/content/SMA12-4671/TIP54.pdf

11

Social Factors and Intimacy

The impacts of chronic pain extend beyond the individual and include family members, friends, and even coworkers. For the patient, the social impacts of chronic pain can be some of the most burdensome. Individuals may feel a loss to personal identity when chronic pain prevents them from participating fully in valued life pursuits and roles—roles that typically involve relationships with others. Lack of satisfaction with roles and responsibilities is an important contributor to emotional distress in chronic pain (Sturgeon, Dixon, Darnall, & Mackey, 2015). For example, parents may experience grief and guilt when they are unable to parent their child as they used to and are missing their child's school and life events. Participating fully in the family's daily life activities and delivering care to others are often important ways one expresses love and derives satisfaction—through acts of giving of oneself. Becoming the recipient of caregiving—rather than being the caregiver to others—can be uncomfortable and distressing.

http://dx.doi.org/10.1037/0000104-012
Psychological Treatment for Patients With Chronic Pain, by B. D. Darnall

Pain waxes and wanes, leaving individuals unsure about how they will feel from one day to the next or even moment to moment. Virtually everyone with chronic pain has had severe pain while in a social situation, leaving them feeling somewhat trapped and wishing they were at home instead. The unpredictability of pain can lead individuals to avoid making social plans out of fear that they will be forced to cancel them yet again. Over time, friends may become distant, and individuals may find themselves feeling alone with their pain. Pain may be poorly understood by friends, coworkers, and family members, further compounding a sense of isolation. The invisibility of chronic pain creates special social challenges, where it is unknown, overlooked, or forgotten by those who do not live with it, or individuals may hear unhelpful statements such as, "You don't look like you have chronic pain."

Individuals who are unable to work because of pain may experience a tremendous loss of perceived self-worth because they are no longer contributing to the social whole in a way that is meaningful to them. They may also simply miss the social contacts of their workdays and the positive reinforcement they gained for doing their job well.

Social stress can amplify pain. Research has suggested that feelings of social rejection or loss activate the same regions of the brain associated with physical pain (Eisenberger, 2012a, 2012b). In addition, social stress has been linked to greater pain sensitivity in healthy women and women with fibromyalgia (Crettaz et al., 2013).

Susan's story in Chapter 9 illustrates how social factors and desire to maintain social roles may lead patients to engage in behaviors that counterproductively worsen pain and function. Susan's story also illustrates the importance of addressing social factors within the context of psychobehavioral treatment for chronic pain. I have long said that "pain is what gets people in my door, and then we begin focusing on the rest of their life." Although it is a simple sound bite, there is truth to it. Chronic pain requires that individuals make adjustments in their relationships with themselves and other people. Often these adjustments include challenges. Patients learn to become exquisitely aware of what their true needs are, and they must communicate and recalibrate old patterns in relationships and behavior that are no longer sustainable within the context of their chronic pain.

PROBLEMATIC FAMILY DYNAMICS: WHEN HELPING IS NO LONGER HELPFUL

As you have heard throughout the book, helping patients actively engage in the self-management of their pain and helping them adopt a rehabilitation mentality and approach is essential for sustained progress. Family dynamics can sometimes impede progress with pain management and recovery (McCracken, 2005; Miró, de la Vega, Gertz, Jensen, & Engel, 2017; Rosen, Bergeron, Glowacka, Delisle, & Baxter, 2012). For instance, a family member may encourage the patient to adopt a sick role and to rest. The family member may rush to help the patient in nonessential ways, thereby contributing to his or her dependency and disability. Such "solicitous" dynamics may be well-intentioned but ultimately do not help patients gain independence or self-efficacy in their ability to manage their pain and life circumstances. In the case of adolescents and young adults, overly solicitous parent dynamics may enable a "failure-to-launch" scenario in which the individual remains dependent on parents while avoiding the rehabilitation-focused treatments that would allow him or her to progress to the next life stage and independence. Parent guilt may underlie solicitous behavior toward their teen or young adult child. In these cases, unconscious secondary gain—on the part of the patient and family members—may also be playing an important role in maintaining cycles of dependency and disability.

PHYSICAL INTIMACY AND SEXUALITY

For many reasons, chronic pain may negatively affect physical intimacy and sexual activity. Pelvic pain conditions and female-specific pain conditions are particularly prone to sexual interference because the pain condition often includes genital pain (Bois, Bergeron, Rosen, McDuff, & Grégoire, 2013). But all types of chronic pain, such as migraine or back pain, are prone to pain-related sexual interference. Some individuals may find that sexual intercourse causes their pain to worsen. Others may simply have low libido due to pain, fatigue, depression, medications, or other medical conditions.

Individuals with chronic pain may worry about how their lack of sexual intimacy is affecting their spouse or partner. It can be helpful to assess the sexual impacts of pain, as well as the patient's motivation to improve the situation. Assess for other relationship factors that may be maintaining a low libido, such as poor communication or anger. Individual and couples therapy may explore ways to improve physical intimacy, even in the absence of sexual intercourse. Finally, long-term opioids reduce testosterone and can cause erectile dysfunction in men and lower sexual desire in women (Cepeda, Zhu, Vorsanger, & Eichenbaum, 2015; Daniell, 2002, 2008). Hormonal supplementation and/or stopping opioids may restore libido and sexual function.

SOCIAL FACTORS IN CHRONIC PAIN: ASSESSMENT AND TREATMENT

- Assess for the social impacts of chronic pain.
- Improved communication about pain can benefit current relationships.
- Helping patients reengage socially is an important aspect of pain treatment and recovery.
- Evaluate for solicitous family dynamics that may be impeding progress.
- Family therapy may assist with supportive boundary setting and shifting family dynamics to optimize the health and independence of the patient.
- Encourage the patient to set goals to reengage socially in ways that are achievable and meaningful to them.
- Engage the family in understanding more about pain and how it is best treated. Family members can learn how best to support their loved ones who have pain.
- Family therapy may be a helpful treatment approach to consider.
- A sex or couples therapist may help address intimacy challenges.

SOCIAL ENGAGEMENT OPTIONS FOR INDIVIDUALS WITH CHRONIC PAIN

- Volunteer. Even if one cannot maintain a regular work schedule, most individuals can volunteer from time to time. Giving to others nourishes the desire to contribute, and it allows one to receive positive social feedback.

- Online chronic pain support groups may be used.
- Free, local, peer-led support groups sponsored by the American Chronic Pain Association (ACPA; https://theacpa.org) exist in almost every state. If one does not exist locally, you may contact the ACPA if you are interested in hosting one. Socializing with peers with chronic pain may provide comfort and understanding, and peers can learn from each other.
- Cognitive behavioral therapy for pain groups, walking clubs, gentle yoga classes, and chronic pain self-management courses allow people to live beyond their pain while being social.

KEY POINTS

- Some of the most difficult aspects of chronic pain involve how it alters one's social roles and participation in social activities.
- Unhealthy social dynamics can serve to worsen pain and dependency or "sick role" within the family. Proper treatment for chronic pain includes providing pain education to family members and helping everyone distinguish between supporting their loved one and enabling disability.
- Restoring or establishing a meaningful and healthy social connection is an important aspect of psychobehavioral treatment for pain.
- Group evidence-based psychobehavioral treatments for chronic pain can provide therapeutic peer support.

RESOURCES

Dueñas, M., Ojeda, B., Salazar, A., Mico, J. A., & Failde, I. (2016). A review of chronic pain impact on patients, their social environment and the health care system. *Journal of Pain Research*, *9*, 457–467. Retrieved from https://www.ncbi.nlm.nih.gov/pmc/articles/PMC4935027/

12

Summary, Future Directions, Conclusions

G reater interest in and need for low-risk nonopioid treatments is spurring increased interest in psychobehavioral approaches to treat pain. More than 40 years of scientific evidence supports psychobehavioral treatment for chronic pain. Although new pain research continues to elucidate important psychobehavioral targets for relief, core tenets of chronic pain relief remain unchanged. The patient remains the most important person on their pain care team because it is the integration of pain management strategies into their daily lives that will gain them the best results. Best pain care involves a comprehensive biopsychosocial approach and includes psychosocial and movement therapies.

As a mental health professional, you play a vitally important "boots-on-the-ground" role in helping to shift your clients' perception away from a biomedical perspective about their pain treatment. By educating your patients about the role of psychology in changing the pain experience

http://dx.doi.org/10.1037/0000104-013
Psychological Treatment for Patients With Chronic Pain, by B. D. Darnall
Copyright © 2019 by the American Psychological Association. All rights reserved.

and treating pain properly (vs. simply "coping" with pain), you will provide a tremendous service. In working with patients with pain, our most important roles include validating their experience of pain, providing education about what pain is and why psychology matters, and empowering them with the resources and tools they need to reduce their suffering. In doing so, we help them to reduce reliance on doctors, pills, and family members and facilitate greater independence to self-manage pain, symptoms, and their lives.

Although there is a great need for psychologists to become better educated in treating chronic pain, novel treatment approaches such as Internet-based options, pain management apps, and brief, targeted therapies are paving the way to better meet the comprehensive pain treatment needs of millions of Americans who seek relief from persistent pain. Social media provides resources for patients to receive education and support from peers and national organizations, including patient e-mail listservs, Twitter groups, Facebook pages dedicated to chronic pain patient groups and treatments, and online support groups. Despite perennial barriers to health insurance and health care, it is easier than ever to receive information, support, and online resources.

Future directions may include the broad integration of free and low-cost resources into health care, including

- basic pain education (see Resources, videos),
- education for patients and providers on best pain care (see Resources, PainToolkit.org),
- relaxation response training in general medical practices and pain practices with biomedical treatment approaches, and
- American Chronic Pain Association free peer-led support groups.

Such resources mitigate or eliminate many current barriers that exist for psychosocial pain care and may provide a minimal level of intervention that can be scaled with low burden.

Additional future directions for the field include improving education for physicians and medical professionals in the biopsychosocial treatment model of pain and helping clinics and health care organizations integrate pain psychology treatment programs into care pathways. Finally, better training in pain is needed at all levels of psychology education (under-graduate, graduate, postgraduate, and continuing education). As the need for biopsychosocial treatment continues to grow, the field of psychology has the opportunity to develop and lead national programs and solutions that, in addressing the full definition of pain, shepherd psychology to the forefront of clinical, educational, policy, and scientific research efforts that target the prevention and treatment of pain and suffering.

Resources

Websites and Articles

The Pain Toolkit website (https://www.paintoolkit.org/) offers a wealth of pain self-management resources for free or for nominal print cost. The website includes resources for patients, with specific download-able resources for health care clinicians (see https://www.paintoolkit.org/resources/for-professionals).

The Canadian Institute for the Relief of Pain and Disability (http://www.cirpd.org) provides excellent free, live, and archived hour-long webinars on various topics related to pain and relief. For example, the following webinar by Beth Darnall:

Work Wellness and Disability Prevention Institute. (2017, May 17). *Reducing catastrophizing to prevent and treat chronic pain* [Webinar]. Retrieved from http://cirpd.org/Webinars/Pages/Webinar.aspx?wbID=151

This resource list includes the resources from each chapter as well as additional ones.

The National Pain Strategy:

NIH Interagency Pain Research Coordinating Committee. (2015). *National pain strategy: A comprehensive population health-level strategy for pain.* Retrieved from https://iprcc.nih.gov/sites/default/files/HHSNational_Pain_Strategy_508C.pdf

Federal Pain Research Strategy Overview:

NIH Interagency Pain Research Coordinating Committee. (2017). *Federal pain research strategy overview.* Retrieved from https://iprcc.nih.gov/Federal-Pain-Research-Strategy/Overview

A National Center for Biotechnology Information open access article (https://www.ncbi.nlm.nih.gov/pmc/articles/PMC4758272/):

Darnall, B. D., Scheman, J., Davin, S., Burns, J. W., Murphy, J. L., Wilson, A. C., . . . Mackey, S. (2016). Pain psychology: A global needs assessment and national call to action. *Pain Medicine, 17,* 250–263. http://dx.doi.org/10.1093/pm/pnv095

The scientific and ethical imperative to include psychology in pain research and treatment:

Darnall B. (2018). To treat pain, study people in all their complexity. *Nature, 557,* 7. http://dx.doi.org/10.1038/d41586-018-04994-5

Darnall, B. D., Carr, D. B., & Schatman, M. E. (2017). Pain psychology and the biopsychosocial model of pain treatment: Ethical imperatives and social responsibility. *Pain Medicine, 18,* 1413–1415. http://dx.doi.org/10.1093/pm/pnw166

A free guide on the role of psychologists in managing pain (with contributions from D. Bruns and R. Kerns):

American Psychological Association Help Center. *Managing chronic pain: How psychologists can help with pain management.* Retrieved from http://www.apa.org/helpcenter/pain-management.pdf

Discussion of the neurobiology of the psychological dimensions of chronic pain:

Bushnell, M. C., Čeko, M., & Low, L. A. (2013). Cognitive and emotional control of pain and its disruption in chronic pain. *Nature Reviews Neuroscience, 14,* 502–511. http://dx.doi.org/10.1038/nrn3516

Posttraumatic stress disorder (PTSD) clinical checklist:

U.S. Department of Veterans Affairs. (2017). *PTSD checklist for* DSM–5 *(PCL-5).* Retrieved from https://www.ptsd.va.gov/professional/assessment/adult-sr/ptsd-checklist.asp

Measure and scoring: PTSD CheckList—Civilian Version (PCL-C). Available at https://www.mirecc.va.gov/docs/visn6/3_PTSD_CheckList_and_Scoring.pdf

Neurobiology of pain and PTSD (review):

Scioli-Salter, E. R., Forman, D. E., Otis, J. D., Gregor, K., Valovski, I., & Rasmusson, A. M. (2015). The shared neuroanatomy and neurobiology of comorbid chronic pain and PTSD: Therapeutic implications. *The Clinical Journal of Pain, 31,* 363–374. http://dx.doi.org/10.1097/AJP.0000000000000115

PTSD and substance use disorder (free PubMed Central article):

Berenz, E. C., & Coffey, S. F. (2012). Treatment of co-occurring posttraumatic stress disorder and substance use disorders. *Current Psychiatry Reports, 14,* 469–477. http://dx.doi.org/10.1007/s11920-012-0300-0

Pediatric chronic pain:

Palermo, T. M., Valrie, C. R., & Carlson, C. W. (2014). Family and parent influences on pediatric chronic pain. *American Psychologist, 69,* 142–152. http://dx.doi.org/10.1037/a0035216

An overview of psychological treatments for chronic pain:

Sturgeon, J. A. (2014). Psychological therapies for the management of chronic pain. *Psychology Research and Behavior Management, 7,* 115–124. http://dx.doi.org/10.2147/PRBM.S44762

Psychological treatments and pain neurophysiology (open access):

Flor, H. (2014). Psychological pain intervention and neurophysiology: Implications for a mechanism-based approach. *American Psychologist, 69,* 188–196. Retrieved from http://www.apa.org/pubs/journals/releases/amp-a0035254.pdf

Cognitive behavioral therapy (CBT) for chronic pain (open access):

Ehde, D. M., Dillworth, T. M., & Turner, J. A. (2014). Cognitive behavioral therapy for individuals with chronic pain: Efficacy, innovations and directions for future research. *American Psychologist, 69,* 153–166. https://www.apa.org/pubs/ journals/releases/amp-a0035747.pdf

Acceptance and commitment therapy and mindfulness for chronic pain (open access):

McCracken, L. M., & Vowles, K. E. (2014). Acceptance and commitment therapy and mindfulness for chronic pain: Model, process, and progress. *American Psychologist, 69,* 178–187. http://www.apa.org/pubs/journals/releases/amp-a0035623.pdf

Hypnosis (open access):

Jensen, M. P., & Patterson, D. R. (2014). Hypnotic approaches for chronic pain management: Clinical implications of recent research findings. *American Psychologist, 69,* 167–177. http://www.apa.org/pubs/journals/releases/ampa0035644.pdf

Opioid abuse (free download):

Volkow, N. D., & McLellan, A. T. (2016). Opioid abuse in chronic pain— Misconceptions and mitigation strategies. *New England Journal of Medicine, 374,* 1253–1263. Available at http://www.nejm.org/doi/pdf/10.1056/ NEJMra1507771

Older adults (open access):

Molton, I. R., & Terrill, A. L. (2014). Overview of persistent pain in older adults. *American Psychologist, 69,* 197–207. Available at http://www.apa.org/pubs/ journals/releases/amp-a0035794.pdf

Racial and ethnic disparities (open access):

Tait, R. C., & Chibnall, J. T. (2014). Racial/ethnic disparities in the assessment and treatment of pain: Psychosocial perspectives. *American Psychologist, 69,* 131–141. Retrieved from http://www.apa.org/pubs/journals/releases/amp-a0035204.pdf

Chronic pain and social factors (open access):

Dueñas, M., Ojeda, B., Salazar, A., Mico, J. A., & Failde, I. (2016). A review of chronic pain impact on patients, their social environment and the health care system. *Journal of Pain Research, 9,* 457–467. Retrieved from https:// www.ncbi.nlm.nih.gov/pmc/articles/PMC4935027/

Treatment Manuals

The Pain Catastrophizing Scale User Manual (with cited scientific background):

Sullivan, M. J. L. (2009). *The Pain Catastrophizing Scale user manual.* Retrieved from http://sullivan-painresearch.mcgill.ca/pdf/pcs/PCSManual_English.pdf

Free evidence-based treatment manual used by the Veterans Health Administration for CBT for pain:

Murphy, J. L., McKellar, J. D., Raffa, S. D., Clark, M. E., Kerns, R. D., Karlin, B. E. (2014). *Cognitive behavioral therapy for chronic pain: Therapist manual.* Retrieved from https://www.va.gov/PAINMANAGEMENT/docs/CBT-CP_Therapist_Manual.pdf

Free literacy-adapted CBT manuals for chronic pain. Beverly Thorn, PhD, has a wealth of resources available online, including a free pain-CBT workbook for clients as well as therapist scripts: http://pmt.ua.edu/publications.html

Group cognitive therapy for chronic pain instructional manual:

Thorn, B. E. (2017). *Cognitive therapy for chronic pain: A step-by-step guide* (2nd ed.). New York, NY: Guilford Press.

Therapist book for ACT:

Dahl, J., Wilson, K., Luciano, C., & Hayes, S. (2005). *Acceptance and commitment therapy for chronic pain.* Oakland, CA: Context Press.

RESOURCES FOR PEOPLE LIVING WITH PAIN

Organizations and Online Resources

- The American Chronic Pain Association (http://theacpa.org) is dedicated to peer support and education for individuals with chronic pain and their families so that these individuals may live more fully in spite of their pain. Their website includes free pain management tools (print and electronic), local support group information, and a resource guide for chronic pain treatments.

- The Pain Toolkit (https://www.paintoolkit.org/) is an award-winning organization whose website offers a wealth of pain self-management resources for free or for nominal print cost (e.g., $2). Developed by a peer with lived experience in successful pain management.

- Pain Research News (http://relief.news) is a pain science roundup of current findings and breaking news in the world of pain research and treatment.

Patient Books

ACT based:

Dahl, J., Hayes, S. C., & Lundgren, T. (2006). *Living beyond your pain: Using acceptance and commitment therapy to ease chronic pain.* Oakland, CA: New Harbinger.

CBT based:

Lewandowski, M. (2006). *The chronic pain care workbook.* Reno, NV: Lucky Bat Books.

Turk, D. W., & Winter, F. (2006). *The pain survival guide: How to reclaim your life.* Washington, DC: American Psychological Association.

The following two resources include a guided binaural relaxation audio file and/or CD:

Darnall, B. (2014). *Less pain, fewer pills: Avoid the dangers of prescription opioids and gain control over chronic pain.* Boulder, CO: Bull Publishing Company.

Darnall, B. (2016). *The opioid-free pain relief kit: 10 simple steps to ease your pain.* Boulder, CO: Bull Publishing Company.

Pain science (pain education):

Butler, D., & Moseley, G. L. (2003). *Explain pain.* Adelaide, Australia: Noigroup.

Chronic pain self-management:

Caudill, M. (2016). *Managing pain before it manages you.* New York, NY: Guilford Press.

Kopf, A., & Patel, N. B. (Eds.). (2010). *Guide to pain management in low-resource settings.* Seattle, WA: International Association for the Treatment of Pain. Retrieved from https://s3.amazonaws.com/rdcms-iasp/files/production/public/Content/ContentFolders/Publications2/FreeBooks/Guide_to_Pain_Management_in_Low-Resource_Settings.pdf

LeFort, S., Webster, L., Lorig, K., Holman, H., Sobel, D., Laurent, D., González, V., & Minor, M. (2015). *Living a healthy life with chronic pain.* Boulder, CO: Bull Publishing Company.

Mindfulness-based stress reduction:

Kabat-Zinn, J. (2013). *Full catastrophe living: Using the wisdom of your body and mind to face stress, pain, and illness.* New York, NY: Penguin Random House.

Hypnosis:

Spiegel, H., & Spiegel, D. (2004). *Trance and treatment: Clinical uses of hypnosis* (2nd ed.). Washington, DC: American Psychiatric Association Publishing.

Integrative pain management:

Stein, T. (2016). *The everything guide to integrative pain management: Conventional and alternative therapies for managing pain.* Avon, MA: Adams Media.

Sleep—patient workbook:

Carney, C., & Manber, R. (2009). *Quiet your mind and get to sleep: Solutions to insomnia for those with depression, anxiety or chronic pain.* Oakland, CA: New Harbinger.

Videos

In a brief video (3:35), a patient describes her successful experience with group CBT for chronic low back pain. This video may be particularly useful for patients who are ambivalent about pain psychology:

Stanford Medicine [Stanford Pain Medicine]. (2017, June 25). *Tina CBT testimonial* [Video file]. Retrieved from http://bit.ly/cbtforchronicpain

An excellent quick resource for patients:

GP Access and Hunter Integrated Pain Service [Painaustralia]. (2012, July 16). *Understanding pain: What to do about it in less than five minutes* [Video file]. Retrieved from https://www.youtube.com/watch?v=RWMKucuejIs

This link contains about 50 different videos on pain self-management, with separate categories for patients and medical providers: https://www.paintoolkit.org/resources/useful-videos

Brief videos (less than 5 minutes) that demystify pain:

Bruns, D. [healthpsych.com]. (2017, October 5). *Riddles of pain* [Video files]. Retrieved from http://bit.ly/pain_riddles

The following video (22:48) describes the biopsychosocial nature of pain:

Bruns, D. [healthpsych.com]. (2017, January 15). *Pain explained part 1* [Video file]. Retrieved from http://bit.ly/pain_explained

The following video (6:53) describes pain catastrophizing:

Darnall, B. [Stanford Pain Medicine]. (2015, August 3). *Stanford's Beth Darnall, PhD on pain catastrophizing* [Video file]. Retrieved from https://www.youtube.com/watch?v=fnNAF4EPFzc

The following video (37:42) describes how you can access your personal tools:

Darnall, B. [Stanford Pain Medicine]. (2015, September 21). *Stanford's Beth Darnall, PhD on "unlocking the medicine box in your mind"* [Video file]. Retrieved from https://www.youtube.com/watch?v=GeqLbJRci1Y

Retrain Pain Foundation offers several 1-minute educational videos on pain and how to manage it (see https://www.retrainpain.org/).

Treatment Resource Guides

Chronic pain treatment resource guide:

The American Chronic Pain Association publishes an annual consumer guide, which may be useful for patients and psychologists alike:

American Chronic Pain Association. (2018). *ACPA resource guide to chronic pain management: An integrated guide to medical, interventional, behavioral, pharmacologic and rehabilitation therapies.* Retrieved from https://www.theacpa.org/wp-content/uploads/2018/03/ACPA_Resource_Guide_2018-Final-v2.pdf

PTSD and chronic pain resource guide:

A free resource guide for health care providers on the comorbid experience of posttraumatic stress disorder and pain:

DeCarvalho, L. T. (2016). *The experience of chronic pain and PTSD: A guide for health care providers.* Retrieved from https://www.ptsd.va.gov/professional/co-occurring/chronic-pain-ptsd-providers.asp

Substance use disorders:

Substance Abuse and Mental Health Services Administration. (2012). *Managing chronic pain in adults with or in recovery from substance use disorders.* Retrieved from https://store.samhsa.gov/shin/content/SMA12-4671/TIP54.pdf

Behavioral health therapist locators:

Acceptance and commitment therapy. Locate an ACT therapist anywhere in the world: https://contextualscience.org/civicrm/profile?gid=17&reset=1&force=1

Online Mindfulness-Based Stress Reduction, Mindfulness, Meditation, and Relaxation Resources

Free online 8-week mindfulness-based stress reduction (MBSR) course: https://palousemindfulness.com/

Free guided meditations (in English and Spanish), MBSR videos, and resources from the University of California, Los Angeles are available online (see http://marc.ucla.edu/mindful-meditations).

Free mindfulness app:

MindApps. (2018). The Mindfulness App (Version 4.7.004) [Mobile application software]. Retrieved from https://www.apple.com/itunes

Free mobile relaxation app (from the Department of Defense):

National Center for Telehealth & Technology. (2016). Breathe2Relax (Version 1.7) [Mobile application software]. Retrieved from http://t2health.dcoe.mil/apps/breathe2relax

Headspace Guided Meditation (visit https://www.headspace.com/ for details), available for purchase at https://www.apple.com/itunes

Mindful.org offers a wealth of mindfulness information, videos, and tips on how to get started (see https://www.mindful.org/meditation/mindfulness-getting-started/).

A mindfulness meditation website, 10% Happier, hosted by Dan Harris and Joseph Goldstein: http://www.10percenthappier.com/mindfulness-meditation-the-basics/

A free meditation app with over 8,000 guided meditations (https://insighttimer.com/):

Insight Network Inc. (2018). Insight Timer—Meditation App (Version 12.2.32) [Mobile application software]. Retrieved from https://www.apple.com/itunes

An hour-long podcast designed to facilitate sleep:

Ackerman, D. (Creator). (2013, October 18). *Sleep with me* [Audio podcast]. Retrieved from http://www.sleepwithmepodcast.com/

Biofeedback

Locate a certified biofeedback therapist at http://www.bcia.org. Go to the "Find a Practitioner" tab and conduct a radius search based on the client's zip code.

Biofeedback for migraine. The American Migraine Foundation: https://americanmigrainefoundation.org/understanding-migraine/biofeedback-and-relaxation-training-for-headaches/

Sherman, R. A., & Hermann, C. (n.d.). *Clinical efficacy of psychophysiological assessments and biofeedback intervention for chronic pain disorders other than head area pain.* Retrieved from https://www.aapb.org/files/public/ReviewOfBFBForPain.pdf

Pain Management Audio File

Binaural audio file (CD or MP3; 20 minutes; $6) includes diaphragmatic breathing, progressive muscle relaxation, and autogenic training (https://www.bullpub.com/catalog/Enhanced-Pain-Management-Binaural-Relaxation-CD):

Darnall, B. (2014). Enhanced pain management [Audio CD or MP3]. Boulder, CO: Bull Publishing Company.

Cognitive Behavioral Therapy Sleep App

Free app that provides sleep education and guides users to develop positive habits that improve sleep:

U.S. Department of Veterans Affairs. (2018). CBT-i Coach (Version 2.3) [Mobile application software]. Retrieved from https://www.apple.com/itunes

References

Abbott, A. D., Tyni-Lenné, R., & Hedlund, R. (2011). Leg pain and psychological variables predict outcome 2–3 years after lumbar fusion surgery. *European Spine Journal, 20,* 1626–1634. http://dx.doi.org/10.1007/s00586-011-1709-6

Affleck, G., Urrows, S., Tennen, H., Higgins, P., & Abeles, M. (1996). Sequential daily relations of sleep, pain intensity, and attention to pain among women with fibromyalgia. *Pain, 68,* 363–368. http://dx.doi.org/10.1016/S0304-3959(96)03226-5

Åkerblom, S., Perrin, S., Rivano Fischer, M., & McCracken, L. M. (2017). The impact of PTSD on functioning in patients seeking treatment for chronic pain and validation of the Posttraumatic Diagnostic Scale. *International Journal of Behavioral Medicine, 24,* 249–259. http://dx.doi.org/10.1007/s12529-017-9641-8

Alattar, M. A., & Scharf, S. M. (2009). Opioid-associated central sleep apnea: A case series. *Sleep and Breathing, 13,* 201–206. http://dx.doi.org/10.1007/s11325-008-0221-7

American Chronic Pain Association. (2015). *ACPA resource guide to chronic pain medication and treatment.* Rocklin, CA: Author. Retrieved from https://www.theacpa.org

American Chronic Pain Association. (2017). *ACPA resource guide to chronic pain medication and treatment: An integrated guide to physical, behavioral and pharmacologic therapy.* Rocklin, CA: Author. Retrieved from https://www.theacpa.org

American College of Occupational and Environmental Medicine. (2017). *2017 American College of Occupational and Environmental Medicine (ACOEM) Practice Guidelines for Chronic Pain.* Westminster, CO: Reed Group, Ltd. Retrieved from http://www.MDGuidelines.com

American Pain Society. (2016). *Principles of analgesic use* (7th ed.). Chicago, IL: Author.

American Psychiatric Association. (2013). *Diagnostic and statistical manual of mental disorders* (5th ed.). Washington, DC: Author.

Andreucci, A., Campbell, P., & Dunn, K. M. (2017). Are sleep problems a risk factor for the onset of musculoskeletal pain in children and adolescents? A systematic review. *Sleep, 40*, zsx093. http://dx.doi.org/10.1093/sleep/zsx093

Archer, K. R., Devin, C. J., Vanston, S. W., Koyama, T., Phillips, S. E., George, S. Z., . . . Wegener, S. T. (2016). Cognitive-behavioral-based physical therapy for patients with chronic pain undergoing lumbar spine surgery: A randomized controlled trial. *The Journal of Pain, 17*, 76–89. http://dx.doi.org/10.1016/j.jpain.2015.09.013

Archer, K. R., Seebach, C. L., Mathis, S. L., Riley, L. H., III, & Wegener, S. T. (2014). Early postoperative fear of movement predicts pain, disability, and physical health six months after spinal surgery for degenerative conditions. *The Spine Journal, 14*, 759–767. http://dx.doi.org/10.1016/j.spinee.2013.06.087

Arnold, L. M., Hudson, J. I., Keck, P. E., Jr., Auchenbach, M. B., Javaras, K. N., & Hess, E. V. (2006). Comorbidity of fibromyalgia and psychiatric disorders. *The Journal of Clinical Psychiatry, 67*, 1219–1225. http://dx.doi.org/10.4088/JCP.v67n0807

Asmundson, G. J., & Katz, J. (2009). Understanding the co-occurrence of anxiety disorders and chronic pain: State-of-the-art. *Depression and Anxiety, 26*, 888–901. http://dx.doi.org/10.1002/da.20600

Attal, N., Cruccu, G., Baron, R., Haanpää, M., Hansson, P., Jensen, T. S., Nurmikko, T., & the European Federation of Neurological Societies. (2010). EFNS guidelines on the pharmacological treatment of neuropathic pain: 2010 Revision. *European Journal of Neurology, 17*, 1113–e88. http://dx.doi.org/10.1111/j.1468-1331.2010.02999.x

Bair, M. J., Robinson, R. L., Katon, W., & Kroenke, K. (2003). Depression and pain comorbidity: A literature review. *Archives of Internal Medicine, 163*, 2433–2445. http://dx.doi.org/10.1001/archinte.163.20.2433

Bartley, E. J., & Fillingim, R. B. (2013). Sex differences in pain: A brief review of clinical and experimental findings. *British Journal of Anaesthesia, 111*, 52–58. http://dx.doi.org/10.1093/bja/aet127

Bartley, E. J., King, C. D., Sibille, K. T., Cruz-Almeida, Y., Riley, J. L., III, Glover, T. L., . . . Fillingim, R. B. (2016). Enhanced pain sensitivity among individuals with symptomatic knee osteoarthritis: Potential sex differences in central sensitization. *Arthritis Care & Research, 68*, 472–480. http://dx.doi.org/10.1002/acr.22712

Bingel, U., Wanigasekera, V., Wiech, K., Ni Mhuircheartaigh, R., Lee, M. C., Ploner, M., & Tracey, I. (2011). The effect of treatment expectation on drug efficacy:

Imaging the analgesic benefit of the opioid remifentanil. *Science Translational Medicine, 3,* 70ra14. http://dx.doi.org/10.1126/scitranslmed.3001244

Bois, K., Bergeron, S., Rosen, N. O., McDuff, P., & Grégoire, C. (2013). Sexual and relationship intimacy among women with provoked vestibulodynia and their partners: Associations with sexual satisfaction, sexual function, and pain self-efficacy. *Journal of Sexual Medicine, 10,* 2024–2035. http://dx.doi.org/10.1111/jsm.12210

Bourn, L. E., Sexton, M. B., Porter, K. E., & Rauch, S. A. (2016). Physical activity moderates the association between pain and PTSD in treatment-seeking veterans. *Pain Medicine, 17,* 2134–2141. http://dx.doi.org/10.1093/pm/pnw089

Braden, J. B., Fan, M. Y., Edlund, M. J., Martin, B. C., DeVries, A., & Sullivan, M. D. (2008). Trends in use of opioids by noncancer pain type 2000–2005 among Arkansas Medicaid and HealthCore enrollees: Results from the TROUP study. *The Journal of Pain, 9,* 1026–1035. http://dx.doi.org/10.1016/j.jpain.2008.06.002

Breckenridge, J., & Clark, J. D. (2003). Patient characteristics associated with opioid versus nonsteroidal anti-inflammatory drug management of chronic low back pain. *The Journal of Pain, 4,* 344–350. http://dx.doi.org/10.1016/S1526-5900(03)00638-2

Breivik, H., Collett, B., Ventafridda, V., Cohen, R., & Gallacher, D. (2006). Survey of chronic pain in Europe: Prevalence, impact on daily life, and treatment. *European Journal of Pain, 10,* 287–333. http://dx.doi.org/10.1016/j.ejpain.2005.06.009

Brennan, P. L., Schutte, K. K., & Moos, R. H. (2005). Pain and use of alcohol to manage pain: Prevalence and 3-year outcomes among older problem and non-problem drinkers. *Addiction, 100,* 777–786. http://dx.doi.org/10.1111/j.1360-0443.2005.01074.x

Brinjikji, W., Luetmer, P. H., Comstock, B., Bresnahan, B. W., Chen, L. E., Deyo, R. A., . . . Jarvik, J. G. (2015). Systematic literature review of imaging features of spinal degeneration in asymptomatic populations. *American Journal of Neuroradiology, 36,* 811–816. http://dx.doi.org/10.3174/ajnr.A4173

Bruffaerts, R., Demyttenaere, K., Kessler, R. C., Tachimori, H., Bunting, B., Hu, C., . . . Scott, K. M. (2015). The associations between preexisting mental disorders and subsequent onset of chronic headaches: A worldwide epidemiologic perspective. *The Journal of Pain, 16,* 42–52. http://dx.doi.org/10.1016/j.jpain.2014.10.002

Brydon, L., Edwards, S., Mohamed-Ali, V., & Steptoe, A. (2004). Socioeconomic status and stress-induced increases in interleukin-6. *Brain, Behavior, and Immunity, 18,* 281–290. http://dx.doi.org/10.1016/j.bbi.2003.09.011

Buer, N., & Linton, S. J. (2002). Fear-avoidance beliefs and catastrophizing: Occurrence and risk factor in back pain and ADL in the general population. *Pain, 99,* 485–491. http://dx.doi.org/10.1016/S0304-3959(02)00265-8

Burns, J. W., Day, M. A., & Thorn, B. E. (2012). Is reduction in pain catastrophizing a therapeutic mechanism specific to cognitive-behavioral therapy for chronic pain? *Translational Behavioral Medicine, 2,* 22–29. http://dx.doi.org/10.1007/s13142-011-0086-3

Burns, J. W., Glenn, B., Bruehl, S., Harden, R. N., & Lofland, K. (2003). Cognitive factors influence outcome following multidisciplinary chronic pain treatment: A replication and extension of a cross-lagged panel analysis. *Behaviour Research and Therapy, 41,* 1163–1182. http://dx.doi.org/10.1016/S0005-7967(03)00029-9

Burns, J. W., Kubilus, A., Bruehl, S., Harden, R. N., & Lofland, K. (2003). Do changes in cognitive factors influence outcome following multidisciplinary treatment for chronic pain? A cross-lagged panel analysis. *Journal of Consulting and Clinical Psychology, 71,* 81–91. http://dx.doi.org/10.1037/0022-006X.71.1.81

Burris, J. L., Cyders, M. A., de Leeuw, R., Smith, G. T., & Carlson, C. R. (2009). Posttraumatic stress disorder symptoms and chronic orofacial pain: An empirical examination of the mutual maintenance model. *Journal of Orofacial Pain, 23,* 243–252.

Burton, A. K., Tillotson, K. M., Main, C. J., & Hollis, S. (1995). Psychosocial predictors of outcome in acute and subchronic low back trouble. *Spine, 20,* 722–728. http://dx.doi.org/10.1097/00007632-199503150-00014

Bushnell, M. C., Čeko, M., & Low, L. A. (2013). Cognitive and emotional control of pain and its disruption in chronic pain. *Nature Reviews Neuroscience, 14,* 502–511. http://dx.doi.org/10.1038/nrn3516

Campbell, C. M., & Edwards, R. R. (2012). Ethnic differences in pain and pain management. *Pain Management, 2,* 219–230. http://dx.doi.org/10.2217/pmt.12.7

Carroll, L. J., Cassidy, J. D., & Côté, P. (2003). Factors associated with the onset of an episode of depressive symptoms in the general population. *Journal of Clinical Epidemiology, 56,* 651–658. http://dx.doi.org/10.1016/S0895-4356(03)00118-5

Carroll, L. J., Cassidy, J. D., & Côté, P. (2004). Depression as a risk factor for onset of an episode of troublesome neck and low back pain. *Pain, 107,* 134–139. http://dx.doi.org/10.1016/j.pain.2003.10.009

Casey, P. P., Feyer, A. M., & Cameron, I. D. (2011). Identifying predictors of early non-recovery in a compensation setting: The Whiplash Outcome Study. *Injury, 42,* 25–32. http://dx.doi.org/10.1016/j.injury.2010.07.234

Cepeda, M. S., Zhu, V., Vorsanger, G., & Eichenbaum, G. (2015). Effect of opioids on testosterone levels: Cross-sectional study using NHANES. *Pain Medicine*, *16*, 2235–2242. http://dx.doi.org/10.1111/pme.12843

Cheatle, M. D., & Webster, L. R. (2015). Opioid therapy and sleep disorders: Risks and mitigation strategies. *Pain Medicine*, *16*, S22–S26. http://dx.doi.org/10.1111/pme.12910

Cherkin, D. C., Sherman, K. J., Balderson, B. H., Cook, A. J., Anderson, M. L., Hawkes, R. J., . . . Turner, J. A. (2016). Effect of mindfulness-based stress reduction vs cognitive behavioral therapy or usual care on back pain and functional limitations in adults with chronic low back pain: A randomized clinical trial. *JAMA*, *315*, 1240–1249. http://dx.doi.org/10.1001/jama.2016.2323

Cicero, T. J., Lynskey, M., Todorov, A., Inciardi, J. A., & Surratt, H. L. (2008). Co-morbid pain and psychopathology in males and females admitted to treatment for opioid analgesic abuse. *Pain*, *139*, 127–135. http://dx.doi.org/10.1016/j.pain.2008.03.021

Colloca, L., & Benedetti, F. (2007). Nocebo hyperalgesia: How anxiety is turned into pain. *Current Opinion in Anaesthesiology*, *20*, 435–439. http://dx.doi.org/10.1097/ACO.0b013e3282b972fb

Crettaz, B., Marziniak, M., Willeke, P., Young, P., Hellhammer, D., Stumpf, A., & Burgmer, M. (2013). Stress-induced allodynia—evidence of increased pain sensitivity in healthy humans and patients with chronic pain after experimentally induced psychosocial stress. *PLoS ONE*, *8*, e69460. http://dx.doi.org/10.1371/journal.pone.0069460

Crider, A., Glaros, A. G., & Gevirtz, R. N. (2005). Efficacy of biofeedback-based treatments for temporomandibular disorders. *Applied Psychophysiology and Biofeedback*, *30*, 333–345. http://dx.doi.org/10.1007/s10484-005-8420-5

Cuijpers, P. (2014). Combined pharmacotherapy and psychotherapy in the treatment of mild to moderate major depression? *JAMA Psychiatry*, *71*, 747–748. http://dx.doi.org/10.1001/jamapsychiatry.2014.277

Daniell, H. W. (2002). Hypogonadism in men consuming sustained-action oral opioids. *The Journal of Pain*, *3*, 377–384. http://dx.doi.org/10.1054/jpai.2002.126790

Daniell, H. W. (2008). Opioid endocrinopathy in women consuming prescribed sustained-action opioids for control of nonmalignant pain. *The Journal of Pain*, *9*, 28–36. http://dx.doi.org/10.1016/j.jpain.2007.08.005

Darnall, B. (2014a). *Less pain, fewer pills: Avoid the dangers of prescription opioids and gain control over chronic pain*. Boulder, CO: Bull Publishing Company.

Darnall, B. D. (2014b). Minimize opioids by optimizing pain psychology. *Pain Management*, *4*, 251–253. http://dx.doi.org/10.2217/pmt.14.18

Darnall, B. D., Scheman, J., Davin, S., Burns, J. W., Murphy, J. L., Wilson, A. C., . . . Mackey, S. C. (2016). Pain psychology: A global needs assessment and national call to action. *Pain Medicine, 17*, 250–263. http://dx.doi.org/10.1093/pm/pnv095

Darnall, B. D., & Suarez, E. C. (2009). Sex and gender in psychoneuroimmunology research: Past, present and future. *Brain, Behavior, and Immunity, 23*, 595–604. http://dx.doi.org/10.1016/j.bbi.2009.02.019

Darnall, B. D., Ziadni, M. S., Stieg, R. L., Mackey, I. G., Kao, M.-C., & Flood, P. (2018). Patient-centered prescription opioid tapering in community outpatients with chronic pain. *JAMA Internal Medicine, 178*, 707–708. http://dx.doi.org/10.1001/jamainternmed.2017.8709

Davis, D. A., Luecken, L. J., & Zautra, A. J. (2005). Are reports of childhood abuse related to the experience of chronic pain in adulthood? A meta-analytic review of the literature. *The Clinical Journal of Pain, 21*, 398–405. http://dx.doi.org/10.1097/01.ajp.0000149795.08746.31

Defrin, R., Lahav, Y., & Solomon, Z. (2017). Dysfunctional pain modulation in torture survivors: The mediating effect of PTSD. *The Journal of Pain, 18*, 1–10. http://dx.doi.org/10.1016/j.jpain.2016.09.005

de Jonghe, F., Hendricksen, M., van Aalst, G., Kool, S., Peen, V., Van, R., . . . Dekker, J. (2004). Psychotherapy alone and combined with pharmacotherapy in the treatment of depression. *The British Journal of Psychiatry, 185*, 37–45. http://dx.doi.org/10.1192/bjp.185.1.37

de Jonghe, F., Kool, S., van Aalst, G., Dekker, J., & Peen, J. (2001). Combining psychotherapy and antidepressants in the treatment of depression. *Journal of Affective Disorders, 64*, 217–229. http://dx.doi.org/10.1016/S0165-0327(00)00259-7

Denison, E., Asenlöf, P., & Lindberg, P. (2004). Self-efficacy, fear avoidance, and pain intensity as predictors of disability in subacute and chronic musculoskeletal pain patients in primary health care. *Pain, 111*, 245–252. http://dx.doi.org/10.1016/j.pain.2004.07.001

Derbyshire, S. W., Whalley, M. G., & Oakley, D. A. (2009). Fibromyalgia pain and its modulation by hypnotic and non-hypnotic suggestion: An fMRI analysis. *European Journal of Pain, 13*, 542–550. http://dx.doi.org/10.1016/j.ejpain.2008.06.010

Diener, I., Kargela, M., & Louw, A. (2016). Listening is therapy: Patient interviewing from a pain science perspective. *Physiotherapy Theory and Practice, 32*, 356–367. http://dx.doi.org/10.1080/09593985.2016.1194648

Dimsdale, J. E., Norman, D., DeJardin, D., & Wallace, M. S. (2007). The effect of opioids on sleep architecture. *Journal of Clinical Sleep Medicine, 3*, 33–36.

Dowell, D., Haegerich, T. M., & Chou, R. (2016). *CDC guideline for prescribing opioids for chronic pain—United States, 2016.* Retrieved from https://www.cdc.gov/mmwr/volumes/65/rr/rr6501e1.htm

Edlund, M. J., Martin, B. C., Fan, M. Y., Braden, J. B., Devries, A., & Sullivan, M. D. (2010). An analysis of heavy utilizers of opioids for chronic noncancer pain in the TROUP study. *Journal of Pain and Symptom Management, 40,* 279–289. http://dx.doi.org/10.1016/j.jpainsymman.2010.01.012

Edlund, M. J., Martin, B. C., Fan, M. Y., Devries, A., Braden, J. B., & Sullivan, M. D. (2010). Risks for opioid abuse and dependence among recipients of chronic opioid therapy: Results from the TROUP study. *Drug and Alcohol Dependence, 112,* 90–98. http://dx.doi.org/10.1016/j.drugalcdep.2010.05.017

Edlund, M. J., Steffick, D., Hudson, T., Harris, K. M., & Sullivan, M. (2007). Risk factors for clinically recognized opioid abuse and dependence among veterans using opioids for chronic non-cancer pain. *Pain, 129,* 355–362. http://dx.doi.org/10.1016/j.pain.2007.02.014

Ehde, D. M., Dillworth, T. M., & Turner, J. A. (2014). Cognitive-behavioral therapy for individuals with chronic pain: Efficacy, innovations, and directions for research. *American Psychologist, 69,* 153–166. http://dx.doi.org/10.1037/a0035747

Eisenberger, N. I. (2012a). The neural bases of social pain: Evidence for shared representations with physical pain. *Psychosomatic Medicine, 74,* 126–135. http://dx.doi.org/10.1097/PSY.0b013e3182464dd1

Eisenberger, N. I. (2012b). The pain of social disconnection: Examining the shared neural underpinnings of physical and social pain. *Nature Reviews Neuroscience, 13,* 421–434. http://dx.doi.org/10.1038/nrn3231

Fillingim, R. B. (2000). Sex, gender, and pain: Women and men really are different. *Current Review of Pain, 4,* 24–30. http://dx.doi.org/10.1007/s11916-000-0006-6

Fillingim, R. B. (2015). Biopsychosocial contributions to sex differences in pain. *BJOG, 122,* 769. http://dx.doi.org/10.1111/1471-0528.13337

Fillingim, R. B., King, C. D., Ribeiro-Dasilva, M. C., Rahim-Williams, B., & Riley, J. L., III. (2009). Sex, gender, and pain: A review of recent clinical and experimental findings. *The Journal of Pain, 10,* 447–485. http://dx.doi.org/10.1016/j.jpain.2008.12.001

Finan, P. H., Buenaver, L. F., Bounds, S. C., Hussain, S., Park, R. J., Haque, U. J., . . . Smith, M. T. (2013). Discordance between pain and radiographic severity in knee osteoarthritis: Findings from quantitative sensory testing of central sensitization. *Arthritis and Rheumatism, 65,* 363–372. http://dx.doi.org/10.1002/art.34646

Fletcher, C., Bradnam, L., & Barr, C. (2016). The relationship between knowledge of pain neurophysiology and fear avoidance in people with chronic pain:

A point in time, observational study. *Physiotherapy Theory and Practice, 32,* 271–276. http://dx.doi.org/10.3109/09593985.2015.1138010

Friedrichsdorf, S. J., Giordano, J., Desai Dakoji, K., Warmuth, A., Daughtry, C., & Schulz, C. A. (2016). Chronic pain in children and adolescents: Diagnosis and treatment of primary pain disorders in head, abdomen, muscles and joints. *Children, 3,* 42. http://dx.doi.org/10.3390/children3040042

Gatchel, R. J., McGeary, D. D., McGeary, C. A., & Lippe, B. (2014). Interdisciplinary chronic pain management: Past, present, and future. *American Psychologist, 69,* 119–130. http://dx.doi.org/10.1037/a0035514

Generaal, E., Vogelzangs, N., Penninx, B. W., & Dekker, J. (2017). Insomnia, sleep duration, depressive symptoms, and the onset of chronic multisite musculoskeletal pain. *Sleep, 40,* zsw030. http://dx.doi.org/10.1093/sleep/zsw030

George, S. Z. (2006). Fear: A factor to consider in musculoskeletal rehabilitation. *The Journal of Orthopaedic and Sports Physical Therapy, 36,* 264–266. http://dx.doi.org/10.2519/jospt.2006.0106

George, S. Z., Fritz, J. M., Bialosky, J. E., & Donald, D. A. (2003). The effect of a fear-avoidance-based physical therapy intervention for patients with acute low back pain: Results of a randomized clinical trial. *Spine, 28,* 2551–2560. http://dx.doi.org/10.1097/01.BRS.0000096677.84605.A2

George, S. Z., Wittmer, V. T., Fillingim, R. B., & Robinson, M. E. (2010). Comparison of graded exercise and graded exposure clinical outcomes for patients with chronic low back pain. *The Journal of Orthopaedic and Sports Physical Therapy, 40,* 694–704. http://dx.doi.org/10.2519/jospt.2010.3396

Gerrits, M. M., van Oppen, P., van Marwijk, H. W., Penninx, B. W., & van der Horst, H. E. (2014). Pain and the onset of depressive and anxiety disorders. *Pain, 155,* 53–59. http://dx.doi.org/10.1016/j.pain.2013.09.005

Gerrits, M. M., Vogelzangs, N., van Oppen, P., van Marwijk, H. W., van der Horst, H., & Penninx, B. W. (2012). Impact of pain on the course of depressive and anxiety disorders. *Pain, 153,* 429–436. http://dx.doi.org/10.1016/j.pain.2011.11.001

Gheldof, E. L., Crombez, G., van den Bussche, E., Vinck, J., Van Nieuwenhuyse, A., Moens, G., . . . Vlaeyen, J. W. (2010). Pain-related fear predicts disability, but not pain severity: A path analytic approach of the fear-avoidance model. *European Journal of Pain, 14,* 870.e1–870.e9. http://dx.doi.org/10.1016/j.ejpain.2010.01.003

Glombiewski, J. A., Bernardy, K., & Häuser, W. (2013). Efficacy of EMG- and EEG-biofeedback in fibromyalgia syndrome: A meta-analysis and a systematic review of randomized controlled trials. *Evidence-Based Complementary and Alternative Medicine, 2013,* 962741. http://dx.doi.org/10.1155/2013/962741

Gracely, R. H., Geisser, M. E., Giesecke, T., Grant, M. A., Petzke, F., Williams, D. A., & Clauw, D. J. (2004). Pain catastrophizing and neural responses to pain among persons with fibromyalgia. *Brain, 127*, 835–843. http://dx.doi.org/10.1093/brain/awh098

Grattan, A., Sullivan, M. D., Saunders, K. W., Campbell, C. I., & Von Korff, M. R. (2012). Depression and prescription opioid misuse among chronic opioid therapy recipients with no history of substance abuse. *Annals of Family Medicine, 10*, 304–311. http://dx.doi.org/10.1370/afm.1371

Green, C. R., Anderson, K. O., Baker, T. A., Campbell, L. C., Decker, S., Fillingim, R. B., . . . Vallerand, A. H. (2003). The unequal burden of pain: Confronting racial and ethnic disparities in pain. *Pain Medicine, 4*, 277–294. http://dx.doi.org/10.1046/j.1526-4637.2003.03034.x

Guilleminault, C., Cao, M., Yue, H. J., & Chawla, P. (2010). Obstructive sleep apnea and chronic opioid use. *Lung, 188*, 459–468. http://dx.doi.org/10.1007/s00408-010-9254-3

Harris, R. A. (2014). Chronic pain, social withdrawal, and depression. *Journal of Pain Research, 7*, 555–556. http://dx.doi.org/10.2147/JPR.S71292

Held, F., Le Couteur, D. G., Blyth, F. M., Hirani, V., Naganathan, V., Waite, L. M., . . . Gnjidic, D. (2017). Polypharmacy in older adults: Association rule and frequent-set analysis to evaluate concomitant medication use. *Pharmacological Research, 116*, 39–44. http://dx.doi.org/10.1016/j.phrs.2016.12.018

Helmerhorst, G. T., Vranceanu, A. M., Vrahas, M., Smith, M., & Ring, D. (2014). Risk factors for continued opioid use one to two months after surgery for musculoskeletal trauma. *The Journal of Bone and Joint Surgery, 96*, 495–499. http://dx.doi.org/10.2106/JBJS.L.01406

Hoffman, B. M., Papas, R. K., Chatkoff, D. K., & Kerns, R. D. (2007). Meta-analysis of psychological interventions for chronic low back pain. *Health Psychology, 26*, 1–9. http://dx.doi.org/10.1037/0278-6133.26.1.1

Holbrook, T. L., Hoyt, D. B., Stein, M. B., & Sieber, W. J. (2002). Gender differences in long-term posttraumatic stress disorder outcomes after major trauma: Women are at higher risk of adverse outcomes than men. *The Journal of Trauma, 53*, 882–888. http://dx.doi.org/10.1097/00005373-200211000-00012

Hooten, W. M., Shi, Y., Gazelka, H. M., & Warner, D. O. (2011). The effects of depression and smoking on pain severity and opioid use in patients with chronic pain. *Pain, 152*, 223–229. http://dx.doi.org/10.1016/j.pain.2010.10.045

Hooten, W. M., Townsend, C. O., Bruce, B. K., Schmidt, J. E., Kerkvliet, J. L., Patten, C. A., & Warner, D. O. (2009). Effects of smoking status on immediate treatment outcomes of multidisciplinary pain rehabilitation. *Pain Medicine, 10*, 347–355. http://dx.doi.org/10.1111/j.1526-4637.2008.00494.x

Hubbard, C. S., Khan, S. A., Keaser, M. L., Mathur, V. A., Goyal, M., & Seminowicz, D. A. (2014). Altered brain structure and function correlate with disease severity and pain catastrophizing in migraine patients. *eNeuro, 1*(1). http://dx.doi.org/10.1523/ENEURO.0006-14.2014

Hughes, L. S., Clark, J., Colclough, J. A., Dale, E., & McMillan, D. (2017). Acceptance and commitment therapy (ACT) for chronic pain: A systematic review and meta-analyses. *The Clinical Journal of Pain, 33*, 552–568. http://dx.doi.org/10.1097/AJP.0000000000000425

Institute of Medicine (US) Committee on Advancing Pain Research, Care, and Education. (2011). *Relieving pain in America: A blueprint for transforming prevention, care, education, and research*. Retrieved from https://www.uspainfoundation.org/wp-content/uploads/2016/01/IOM-Full-Report.pdf

International Association for the Study of Pain. (1979). The need of a taxonomy. *Pain, 6*, 247–252.

International Association for the Study of Pain. (2018). *Right to pain relief*. Retrieved from https://www.iasp-pain.org/GlobalYear/RighttoPainRelief

Jahanban-Esfahlan, R., Mehrzadi, S., Reiter, R. J., Seidi, K., Majidinia, M., Baghi, H. B., . . . Sadeghpour, A. (2017). Melatonin in regulation of inflammatory pathways in rheumatoid arthritis and osteoarthritis: Involvement of circadian clock genes. *British Journal of Pharmacology*. Advance online publication. http://dx.doi.org/10.1111/bph.13898

Javaheri, S., & Patel, S. (2017). Opioids cause central and complex sleep apnea in humans and reversal with discontinuation: A plea for detoxification. *Journal of Clinical Sleep Medicine, 13*, 829–833. http://dx.doi.org/10.5664/jcsm.6628

Jiang, Y., Oathes, D., Hush, J., Darnall, B., Charvat, M., Mackey, S., & Etkin, A. (2016). Perturbed connectivity of the amygdala and its subregions with the central executive and default mode networks in chronic pain. *Pain, 157*, 1970–1978. http://dx.doi.org/10.1097/j.pain.0000000000000606

Kalso, E., Edwards, J. E., Moore, R. A., & McQuay, H. J. (2004). Opioids in chronic non-cancer pain: Systematic review of efficacy and safety. *Pain, 112*, 372–380. http://dx.doi.org/10.1016/j.pain.2004.09.019

Karyotaki, E., Smit, Y., Holdt Henningsen, K., Huibers, M. J., Robays, J., de Beurs, D., & Cuijpers, P. (2016). Combining pharmacotherapy and psychotherapy or monotherapy for major depression? A meta-analysis on the long-term effects. *Journal of Affective Disorders, 194*, 144–152. http://dx.doi.org/10.1016/j.jad.2016.01.036

Kessler, R. C., Chiu, W. T., Demler, O., & Walters, E. E. (2005). Prevalence, severity, and comorbidity of 12-month *DSM–IV* disorders in the National Comorbidity Survey Replication. *Archives of General Psychiatry, 62*, 617–627. http://dx.doi.org/10.1001/archpsyc.62.6.617

Khodadadi-Hassankiadeh, N., Dehghan Nayeri, N., Shahsavari, H., Yousefzadeh-Chabok, S., & Haghani, H. (2017). Predictors of post-traumatic stress disorder among victims of serious motor vehicle accidents. *International Journal of Community Based Nursing and Midwifery, 5*, 355–364.

Kim, J., & Parish, A. L. (2017). Polypharmacy and medication management in older adults. *The Nursing Clinics of North America, 52*, 457–468. http://dx.doi.org/10.1016/j.cnur.2017.04.007

Knaster, P., Estlander, A. M., Karlsson, H., Kaprio, J., & Kalso, E. (2016). Diagnosing depression in chronic pain patients: *DSM–IV* major depressive disorder vs. Beck Depression Inventory (BDI). *PLoS ONE, 11*, e0151982. http://dx.doi.org/10.1371/journal.pone.0151982

Kroska, E. B. (2016). A meta-analysis of fear-avoidance and pain intensity: The paradox of chronic pain. *Scandinavian Journal of Pain, 13*, 43–58. http://dx.doi.org/10.1016/j.sjpain.2016.06.011

LaVeist, T. A., Nickerson, K. J., & Bowie, J. V. (2000). Attitudes about racism, medical mistrust, and satisfaction with care among African American and White cardiac patients. *Medical Care Research and Review, 57*, 146–161. http://dx.doi.org/10.1177/1077558700057001S07

Linton, S. J. (2005). Do psychological factors increase the risk for back pain in the general population in both a cross-sectional and prospective analysis? *European Journal of Pain, 9*, 355–361. http://dx.doi.org/10.1016/j.ejpain.2004.08.002

Linton, S. J., Buer, N., Vlaeyen, J., & Hellsing, A. L. (2000). Are fear-avoidance beliefs related to the inception of an episode of back pain? A prospective study. *Psychology & Health, 14*, 1051–1059. http://dx.doi.org/10.1080/08870440008407366

Logan, D. E., Simons, L. E., & Carpino, E. A. (2012). Too sick for school? Parent influences on school functioning among children with chronic pain. *Pain, 153*, 437–443. http://dx.doi.org/10.1016/j.pain.2011.11.004

Lorig, K., & Holman, H. (1993). Arthritis self-management studies: A twelve-year review. *Health Education Quarterly, 20*, 17–28. http://dx.doi.org/10.1177/109019819302000104

Lorig, K., Lubeck, D., Kraines, R. G., Seleznick, M., & Holman, H. R. (1985). Outcomes of self-help education for patients with arthritis. *Arthritis and Rheumatism, 28*, 680–685. http://dx.doi.org/10.1002/art.1780280612

Lorig, K. R. (1982). Arthritis self-management: A patient education program. *Rehabilitation Nursing, 7*, 16–20. http://dx.doi.org/10.1002/j.2048-7940.1982.tb02272.x

Lorig, K. R., Ritter, P. L., Laurent, D. D., & Fries, J. F. (2004). Long-term randomized controlled trials of tailored-print and small-group arthritis self-management interventions. *Medical Care, 42*, 346–354. http://dx.doi.org/10.1097/01.mlr.0000118709.74348.65

Lynch, A. M., Kashikar-Zuck, S., Goldschneider, K. R., & Jones, B. A. (2007). Sex and age differences in coping styles among children with chronic pain. *Journal of Pain and Symptom Management*, *33*, 208–216. http://dx.doi.org/10.1016/j.jpainsymman.2006.07.014

Ma, C., Szeto, G. P., Yan, T., Wu, S., Lin, C., & Li, L. (2011). Comparing biofeedback with active exercise and passive treatment for the management of work-related neck and shoulder pain: A randomized controlled trial. *Archives of Physical Medicine and Rehabilitation*, *92*, 849–858. http://dx.doi.org/10.1016/j.apmr.2010.12.037

Macintyre, P. E., Scott, D. A., Schug, S. A., Visser, E. J., & Walker, S. M. (Eds.). (2010). *Acute pain management: Scientific evidence* (3rd ed.). Retrieved from https://sydney.edu.au/medicine/pmri/pdf/Acute-pain-management-scientific-evidence-third-edition.pdf

Maixner, W., Fillingim, R. B., Williams, D. A., Smith, S. B., & Slade, G. D. (2016). Overlapping chronic pain conditions: Implications for diagnosis and classification. *The Journal of Pain*, *17*, T93–T107. http://dx.doi.org/10.1016/j.jpain.2016.06.002

Marks, R., & Allegrante, J. P. (2005). A review and synthesis of research evidence for self-efficacy-enhancing interventions for reducing chronic disability: Implications for health education practice (Part II). *Health Promotion Practice*, *6*, 148–156. http://dx.doi.org/10.1177/1524839904266792

McCracken, L. M. (2005). Social context and acceptance of chronic pain: The role of solicitous and punishing responses. *Pain*, *113*, 155–159. http://dx.doi.org/10.1016/j.pain.2004.10.004

McLean, S. A., Clauw, D. J., Abelson, J. L., & Liberzon, I. (2005). The development of persistent pain and psychological morbidity after motor vehicle collision: Integrating the potential role of stress response systems into a biopsychosocial model. *Psychosomatic Medicine*, *67*, 783–790. http://dx.doi.org/10.1097/01.psy.0000181276.49204.bb

Melzack, R., & Casey, K. L. (1968). Sensory, motivational, and central control determinants of pain. In D. R. Kenshalo (Ed.), *The skin senses* (pp. 423–439). Springfield, IL: Thomas.

Metikaridis, T. D., Hadjipavlou, A., Artemiadis, A., Chrousos, G., & Darviri, C. (2016). Effect of a stress management program on subjects with neck pain: A pilot randomized controlled trial. *Journal of Back and Musculoskeletal Rehabilitation*, *30*, 23–33. http://dx.doi.org/10.3233/BMR-160709

Mezei, L., & Murinson, B. B. (2011). Pain education in North American medical schools. *The Journal of Pain*, *12*, 1199–1208. http://dx.doi.org/10.1016/j.jpain.2011.06.006

Miller, M. B., Chan, W. S., Boissoneault, J., Robinson, M., Staud, R., Berry, R. B., & McCrae, C. S. (2017). Dynamic daily associations between insomnia symptoms and alcohol use in adults with chronic pain. *Journal of Sleep Research*. Advance online publication. http://dx.doi.org/10.1111/jsr.12604

Mills, P. J., von Känel, R., Norman, D., Natarajan, L., Ziegler, M. G., & Dimsdale, J. E. (2007). Inflammation and sleep in healthy individuals. *Sleep, 30*, 729–735. http://dx.doi.org/10.1093/sleep/30.6.729

Miró, J., de la Vega, R., Gertz, K. J., Jensen, M. P., & Engel, J. M. (2017). The role of perceived family social support and parental solicitous responses in adjustment to bothersome pain in young people with physical disabilities. *Disability and Rehabilitation*. Advance online publication. http://dx.doi.org/10.1080/09638288.2017.1400594

Mogri, M., Khan, M. I. A., Grant, B. J. B., & Mador, M. J. (2008). Central sleep apnea induced by acute ingestion of opioids. *Chest, 133*, 1484–1488. http://dx.doi.org/10.1378/chest.07-1891

Montgomery, G. H., DuHamel, K. N., & Redd, W. H. (2000). A meta-analysis of hypnotically induced analgesia: How effective is hypnosis? *International Journal of Clinical and Experimental Hypnosis, 48*, 138–153. http://dx.doi.org/10.1080/00207140008410045

Morasco, B. J., Turk, D. C., Donovan, D. M., & Dobscha, S. K. (2013). Risk for prescription opioid misuse among patients with a history of substance use disorder. *Drug and Alcohol Dependence, 127*, 193–199. http://dx.doi.org/10.1016/j.drugalcdep.2012.06.032

Morasco, B. J., Yarborough, B. J., Smith, N. X., Dobscha, S. K., Deyo, R. A., Perrin, N. A., & Green, C. A. (2017). Higher prescription opioid dose is associated with worse patient-reported pain outcomes and more health care utilization. *The Journal of Pain, 18*, 437–445. http://dx.doi.org/10.1016/j.jpain.2016.12.004

Moseley, G. L., Nicholas, M. K., & Hodges, P. W. (2004). Does anticipation of back pain predispose to back trouble? *Brain, 127*, 2339–2347. http://dx.doi.org/10.1093/brain/awh248

Murphy, J. L., Clark, M. E., & Banou, E. (2013). Opioid cessation and multidimensional outcomes after interdisciplinary chronic pain treatment. *The Clinical Journal of Pain, 29*, 109–117. http://dx.doi.org/10.1097/AJP.0b013e3182579935

Nguyen, M., Ugarte, C., Fuller, I., Haas, G., & Portenoy, R. K. (2005). Access to care for chronic pain: Racial and ethnic differences. *The Journal of Pain, 6*, 301–314. http://dx.doi.org/10.1016/j.jpain.2004.12.008

Nicholas, M. K., Asghari, A., Blyth, F. M., Wood, B. M., Murray, R., McCabe, R., . . . Overton, S. (2017). Long-term outcomes from training in self-management of chronic pain in an elderly population: A randomized controlled trial. *Pain, 158*, 86–95. http://dx.doi.org/10.1097/j.pain.0000000000000729

NIH Interagency Pain Research Coordinating Committee. (2015). *National pain strategy: A comprehensive population health-level strategy for pain.* Retrieved from https://iprcc.nih.gov/sites/default/files/HHSNational_Pain_Strategy_508C.pdf

Noel, M., Chambers, C. T., McGrath, P. J., Klein, R. M., & Stewart, S. H. (2012). The influence of children's pain memories on subsequent pain experience. *Pain, 153,* 1563–1572. http://dx.doi.org/10.1016/j.pain.2012.02.020

Nugent, S. M., Yarborough, B. J., Smith, N. X., Dobscha, S. K., Deyo, R. A., Green, C. A., & Morasco, B. J. (2018). Patterns and correlates of medical cannabis use for pain among patients prescribed long-term opioid therapy. *General Hospital Psychiatry, 50,* 104–110. http://dx.doi.org/10.1016/j.genhosppsych.2017.11.001

Ohayon, M. M. (2004). Specific characteristics of the pain/depression association in the general population. *The Journal of Clinical Psychiatry, 65,* 5–9.

Öst, L. G. (2014). The efficacy of acceptance and commitment therapy: An updated systematic review and meta-analysis. *Behaviour Research and Therapy, 61,* 105–121. http://dx.doi.org/10.1016/j.brat.2014.07.018

Park, J. Y., & Wu, L. T. (2017). Prevalence, reasons, perceived effects, and correlates of medical marijuana use: A review. *Drug and Alcohol Dependence, 177,* 1–13. http://dx.doi.org/10.1016/j.drugalcdep.2017.03.009

Pavlin, D. J., Sullivan, M. J., Freund, P. R., & Roesen, K. (2005). Catastrophizing: A risk factor for postsurgical pain. *The Clinical Journal of Pain, 21,* 83–90. http://dx.doi.org/10.1097/00002508-200501000-00010

Picavet, H. S., Vlaeyen, J. W., & Schouten, J. S. (2002). Pain catastrophizing and kinesiophobia: Predictors of chronic low back pain. *American Journal of Epidemiology, 156,* 1028–1034. http://dx.doi.org/10.1093/aje/kwf136

Probyn, K., Bowers, H., Mistry, D., Caldwell, F., Underwood, M., Patel, S., . . . Pincus, T., & the CHESS team. (2017). Non-pharmacological self-management for people living with migraine or tension-type headache: A systematic review including analysis of intervention components. *BMJ Open, 7*(8). http://dx.doi.org/10.1136/bmjopen-2017-016670

Rainville, J., Hartigan, C., Martinez, E., Limke, J., Jouve, C., & Finno, M. (2004). Exercise as a treatment for chronic low back pain. *The Spine Journal, 4,* 106–115. http://dx.doi.org/10.1016/S1529-9430(03)00174-8

Ribeiro-Dasilva, M. C., Goodin, B. R., & Fillingim, R. B. (2012). Differences in suprathreshold heat pain responses and self-reported sleep quality between patients with temporomandibular joint disorder and healthy controls. *European Journal of Pain, 16,* 983–993. http://dx.doi.org/10.1002/j.1532-2149.2011.00108.x

Riddle, D. L., Wade, J. B., Jiranek, W. A., & Kong, X. (2010). Preoperative pain catastrophizing predicts pain outcome after knee arthroplasty. *Clinical Orthopaedics and Related Research, 468,* 798–806. http://dx.doi.org/10.1007/s11999-009-0963-y

Roeckel, L. A., Le Coz, G. M., Gavériaux-Ruff, C., & Simonin, F. (2016). Opioid-induced hyperalgesia: Cellular and molecular mechanisms. *Neuroscience, 338,* 160–182. http://dx.doi.org/10.1016/j.neuroscience.2016.06.029

Roh, Y. H., Lee, B. K., Noh, J. H., Oh, J. H., Gong, H. S., & Baek, G. H. (2012). Effect of depressive symptoms on perceived disability in patients with chronic shoulder pain. *Archives of Orthopaedic and Trauma Surgery, 132,* 1251–1257. http://dx.doi.org/10.1007/s00402-012-1545-0

Roh, Y. H., Lee, B. K., Noh, J. H., Oh, J. H., Gong, H. S., & Baek, G. H. (2014). Effect of anxiety and catastrophic pain ideation on early recovery after surgery for distal radius fractures. *The Journal of Hand Surgery, 39,* 2258–2264.e2. http://dx.doi.org/10.1016/j.jhsa.2014.08.007

Roizenblatt, M., Rosa Neto, N. S., Tufik, S., & Roizenblatt, S. (2012). Pain-related diseases and sleep disorders. *Brazilian Journal of Medical and Biological Research, 45,* 792–798. http://dx.doi.org/10.1590/S0100-879X2012007500110

Roizenblatt, S., Rosa Neto, N. S., & Tufik, S. (2011). Sleep disorders and fibromyalgia. *Current Pain and Headache Reports, 15,* 347–357. http://dx.doi.org/10.1007/s11916-011-0213-3

Rosen, N. O., Bergeron, S., Glowacka, M., Delisle, I., & Baxter, M. L. (2012). Harmful or helpful: Perceived solicitous and facilitative partner responses are differentially associated with pain and sexual satisfaction in women with provoked vestibulodynia. *Journal of Sexual Medicine, 9,* 2351–2360. http://dx.doi.org/10.1111/j.1743-6109.2012.02851.x

Rosenberg, J. C., Schultz, D. M., Duarte, L. E., Rosen, S. M., & Raza, A. (2015). Increased pain catastrophizing associated with lower pain relief during spinal cord stimulation: Results from a large post-market study. *Neuromodulation, 18,* 277–284. http://dx.doi.org/10.1111/ner.12287

Rosenbloom, B. N., Khan, S., McCartney, C., & Katz, J. (2013). Systematic review of persistent pain and psychological outcomes following traumatic musculoskeletal injury. *Journal of Pain Research, 6,* 39–51. http://dx.doi.org/10.2147/JPR.S38878

Rosenstiel, A. K., & Keefe, F. J. (1983). The use of coping strategies in chronic low back pain patients: Relationship to patient characteristics and current adjustment. *Pain, 17,* 33–44. http://dx.doi.org/10.1016/0304-3959(83)90125-2

Salas, J., Scherrer, J. F., Schneider, F. D., Sullivan, M. D., Bucholz, K. K., Burroughs, T., . . . Lustman, P. J. (2017). New-onset depression following stable, slow, and rapid rate of prescription opioid dose escalation. *Pain, 158*, 306–312. http://dx.doi.org/10.1097/j.pain.0000000000000763

Saunders, K., Merikangas, K., Low, N. C., Von Korff, M., & Kessler, R. C. (2008). Impact of comorbidity on headache-related disability. *Neurology, 70*, 538–547. http://dx.doi.org/10.1212/01.wnl.0000297192.84581.21

Schappert, S. M., & Rechtsteiner, E. A. (2008). Ambulatory medical care utilization estimates for 2006. *National Health Statistics Reports, Aug 6*, 1–29.

Scherrer, J. F., Salas, J., Schneider, F. D., Bucholz, K. K., Sullivan, M. D., Copeland, L. A., . . . Lustman, P. J. (2017). Characteristics of new depression diagnoses in patients with and without prior chronic opioid use. *Journal of Affective Disorders, 210*, 125–129. http://dx.doi.org/10.1016/j.jad.2016.12.027

Scioli-Salter, E. R., Forman, D. E., Otis, J. D., Gregor, K., Valovski, I., & Rasmusson, A. M. (2015). The shared neuroanatomy and neurobiology of comorbid chronic pain and PTSD: Therapeutic implications. *The Clinical Journal of Pain, 31*, 363–374. http://dx.doi.org/10.1097/AJP.0000000000000115

Segal, J. P., Tresidder, K. A., Bhatt, C., Gilron, I., & Ghasemlou, N. (2018). Circadian control of pain and neuroinflammation. *Journal of Neuroscience Research, 96*, 1002–1020. http://dx.doi.org/10.1002/jnr.24150

Seminowicz, D. A., & Davis, K. D. (2006). Cortical responses to pain in healthy individuals depends on pain catastrophizing. *Pain, 120*, 297–306. http://dx.doi.org/10.1016/j.pain.2005.11.008

Seminowicz, D. A., Shpaner, M., Keaser, M. L., Krauthamer, G. M., Mantegna, J., Dumas, J. A., . . . Naylor, M. R. (2013). Cognitive-behavioral therapy increases prefrontal cortex gray matter in patients with chronic pain. *The Journal of Pain, 14*, 1573–1584. http://dx.doi.org/10.1016/j.jpain.2013.07.020

Severeijns, R., Vlaeyen, J. W., van den Hout, M. A., & Weber, W. E. (2001). Pain catastrophizing predicts pain intensity, disability, and psychological distress independent of the level of physical impairment. *The Clinical Journal of Pain, 17*, 165–172. http://dx.doi.org/10.1097/00002508-200106000-00009

Sharifzadeh, Y., Kao, M. C., Sturgeon, J. A., Rico, T. J., Mackey, S., & Darnall, B. D. (2017). Pain catastrophizing moderates relationships between pain intensity and opioid prescription: Nonlinear sex differences revealed using a learning health system. *Anesthesiology, 127*, 136–146. http://dx.doi.org/10.1097/ALN.0000000000001656

Siebern, A. T., & Manber, R. (2011). New developments in cognitive behavioral therapy as the first-line treatment of insomnia. *Psychology Research and Behavior Management, 4*, 21–28. http://dx.doi.org/10.2147/PRBM.S10041

Sielski, R., Rief, W., & Glombiewski, J. A. (2017). Efficacy of biofeedback in chronic back pain: A meta-analysis. *International Journal of Behavioral Medicine, 24*, 25–41. http://dx.doi.org/10.1007/s12529-016-9572-9

Simpson, T. L., Stappenbeck, C. A., Varra, A. A., Moore, S. A., & Kaysen, D. (2012). Symptoms of posttraumatic stress predict craving among alcohol treatment seekers: Results of a daily monitoring study. *Psychology of Addictive Behaviors, 26*, 724–733. http://dx.doi.org/10.1037/a0027169

Smith, E. M., Pang, H., Cirrincione, C., Fleishman, S., Paskett, E. D., Ahles, T., . . . Shapiro, C. L. (2013). Effect of duloxetine on pain, function, and quality of life among patients with chemotherapy-induced painful peripheral neuropathy: A randomized clinical trial. *JAMA, 309*, 1359–1367. http://dx.doi.org/10.1001/jama.2013.2813

Smith, K. Z., Smith, P. H., Cercone, S. A., McKee, S. A., & Homish, G. G. (2016). Past year non-medical opioid use and abuse and PTSD diagnosis: Interactions with sex and associations with symptom clusters. *Addictive Behaviors, 58*, 167–174. http://dx.doi.org/10.1016/j.addbeh.2016.02.019

Smith, M. T., & Haythornthwaite, J. A. (2004). How do sleep disturbance and chronic pain inter-relate? Insights from the longitudinal and cognitive-behavioral clinical trials literature. *Sleep Medicine Reviews, 8*, 119–132. http://dx.doi.org/10.1016/S1087-0792(03)00044-3

Smith, M. T., & Quartana, P. J. (2010). The riddle of the sphinx: Sleep, pain, and depression. *Sleep Medicine, 11*, 745–746. http://dx.doi.org/10.1016/j.sleep.2010.05.004

Steptoe, A., Hamer, M., & Chida, Y. (2007). The effects of acute psychological stress on circulating inflammatory factors in humans: A review and meta-analysis. *Brain, Behavior, and Immunity, 21*, 901–912. http://dx.doi.org/10.1016/j.bbi.2007.03.011

Stewart, M. O., Karlin, B. E., Murphy, J. L., Raffa, S. D., Miller, S. A., McKeller, J., & Kerns, R. D. (2015). National dissemination of cognitive-behavioral therapy for chronic pain in veterans: Therapist and patient-level outcomes. *The Clinical Journal of Pain, 31*, 722–729. http://dx.doi.org/10.1097/AJP.0000000000000151

Sturgeon, J. A. (2014). Psychological therapies for the management of chronic pain. *Psychology Research and Behavior Management, 7*, 115–124. http://dx.doi.org/10.2147/PRBM.S44762

Sturgeon, J. A., Dixon, E. A., Darnall, B. D., & Mackey, S. C. (2015). Contributions of physical function and satisfaction with social roles to emotional distress in chronic pain: A Collaborative Health Outcomes Information Registry (CHOIR) study. *Pain, 156*, 2627–2633. http://dx.doi.org/10.1097/j.pain.0000000000000313

Sullivan, M. D., Edlund, M. J., Fan, M.-Y., DeVries, A., Braden, J., & Martin, B. C. (2008). Trends in use of opioids for non-cancer pain conditions 2000–2005 in commercial and Medicaid insurance plans: The TROUP study. *Pain, 138*, 440–449. http://dx.doi.org/10.1016/j.pain.2008.04.027

Sullivan, M. D., Edlund, M. J., Fan, M.-Y., DeVries, A., Braden, J., & Martin, B. C. (2010). Risks for possible and probable opioid misuse among recipients of chronic opioid therapy in commercial and Medicaid insurance plans: The TROUP Study. *Pain, 150,* 332–339. http://dx.doi.org/10.1016/j.pain.2010.05.020

Sullivan, M. J. L., Bishop, S. R., & Pivik, J. (1995). The Pain Catastrophizing Scale: Development and validation. *Psychological Assessment, 7,* 524–532. http://dx.doi.org/10.1037/1040-3590.7.4.524

Sullivan, M. J. L., Lynch, M. E., & Clark, A. J. (2005). Dimensions of catastrophic thinking associated with pain experience and disability in patients with neuropathic pain conditions. *Pain, 113,* 310–315. http://dx.doi.org/10.1016/j.pain.2004.11.003

Sumpton, J. E., & Moulin, D. E. (2001). Treatment of neuropathic pain with venlafaxine. *The Annals of Pharmacotherapy, 35,* 557–559. http://dx.doi.org/10.1345/aph.10206

Sun, E. C., Darnall, B. D., Baker, L. C., & Mackey, S. (2016). Incidence of and risk factors for chronic opioid use among opioid-naive patients in the post-operative period. *JAMA Internal Medicine, 176,* 1286–1293. http://dx.doi.org/10.1001/jamainternmed.2016.3298

Sun, E. C., Dixit, A., Humphreys, K., Darnall, B. D., Baker, L. C., & Mackey, S. (2017). Association between concurrent use of prescription opioids and benzodiazepines and overdose: Retrospective analysis. *BMJ, 356,* j760. http://dx.doi.org/10.1136/bmj.j760

Tannenbaum, C. (2013). How to treat the frail elderly: The challenge of multi-morbidity and polypharmacy. *Canadian Urological Association Journal, 7,* 183–185. http://dx.doi.org/10.5489/cuaj.1619

Tepper, D. (2017). Medication overuse headache. *Headache, 57,* 845–846. http://dx.doi.org/10.1111/head.13034

Tesarz, J., Gerhardt, A., Leisner, S., Janke, S., Treede, R. D., & Eich, W. (2015). Distinct quantitative sensory testing profiles in nonspecific chronic back pain subjects with and without psychological trauma. *Pain, 156,* 577–586. http://dx.doi.org/10.1097/01.j.pain.0000460350.30707.8d

Tesarz, J., Leisner, S., Gerhardt, A., Janke, S., Seidler, G. H., Eich, W., & Hartmann, M. (2014). Effects of eye movement desensitization and reprocessing (EMDR) treatment in chronic pain patients: A systematic review. *Pain Medicine, 15,* 247–263. http://dx.doi.org/10.1111/pme.12303

Thakkar, M. M., Sharma, R., & Sahota, P. (2015). Alcohol disrupts sleep homeostasis. *Alcohol, 49,* 299–310. http://dx.doi.org/10.1016/j.alcohol.2014.07.019

Theunissen, M., Peters, M. L., Bruce, J., Gramke, H. F., & Marcus, M. A. (2012). Preoperative anxiety and catastrophizing: A systematic review and meta-analysis of the association with chronic postsurgical pain. *The Clinical Journal of Pain, 28*, 819–841. http://dx.doi.org/10.1097/AJP.0b013e31824549d6

Tighe, P. J., Riley, J. L., III, & Fillingim, R. B. (2014). Sex differences in the incidence of severe pain events following surgery: A review of 333,000 pain scores. *Pain Medicine, 15*, 1390–1404. http://dx.doi.org/10.1111/pme.12498

Tota-Faucette, M. E., Gil, K. M., Williams, D. A., Keefe, F. J., & Goli, V. (1993). Predictors of response to pain management treatment. The role of family environment and changes in cognitive processes. *The Clinical Journal of Pain, 9*, 115–123. http://dx.doi.org/10.1097/00002508-199306000-00006

Tsang, A., Von Korff, M., Lee, S., Alonso, J., Karam, E., Angermeyer, M. C., . . . Watanabe, M. (2008). Common chronic pain conditions in developed and developing countries: Gender and age differences and comorbidity with depression-anxiety disorders. *The Journal of Pain, 9*, 883–891. http://dx.doi.org/10.1016/j.jpain.2008.05.005

Turner, J. A., Anderson, M. L., Balderson, B. H., Cook, A. J., Sherman, K. J., & Cherkin, D. C. (2016). Mindfulness-based stress reduction and cognitive behavioral therapy for chronic low back pain: Similar effects on mindfulness, catastrophizing, self-efficacy, and acceptance in a randomized controlled trial. *Pain, 157*, 2434–2444. http://dx.doi.org/10.1097/j.pain.0000000000000635

Unruh, A. M. (1996). Gender variations in clinical pain experience. *Pain, 65*, 123–167. http://dx.doi.org/10.1016/0304-3959(95)00214-6

Unruh, A. M., Ritchie, J., & Merskey, H. (1999). Does gender affect appraisal of pain and pain coping strategies? *The Clinical Journal of Pain, 15*, 31–40. http://dx.doi.org/10.1097/00002508-199903000-00006

Vissers, M. M., Bussmann, J. B., Verhaar, J. A., Busschbach, J. J., Bierma-Zeinstra, S. M., & Reijman, M. (2012). Psychological factors affecting the outcome of total hip and knee arthroplasty: A systematic review. *Seminars in Arthritis and Rheumatism, 41*, 576–588. http://dx.doi.org/10.1016/j.semarthrit.2011.07.003

Vlaeyen, J. W., & Crombez, G. (1999). Fear of movement/(re)injury, avoidance and pain disability in chronic low back pain patients. *Manual Therapy, 4*, 187–195. http://dx.doi.org/10.1054/math.1999.0199

Vlaeyen, J. W., Crombez, G., & Linton, S. J. (2016). The fear-avoidance model of pain. *Pain, 157*, 1588–1589. http://dx.doi.org/10.1097/j.pain.0000000000000574

Vlaeyen, J. W., & Linton, S. J. (2000). Fear-avoidance and its consequences in chronic musculoskeletal pain: A state of the art. *Pain, 85*, 317–332. http://dx.doi.org/10.1016/S0304-3959(99)00242-0

Volkow, N. D., & McLellan, A. T. (2016). Opioid abuse in chronic pain—Misconceptions and mitigation strategies. *New England Journal of Medicine, 374*, 1253–1263. http://dx.doi.org/10.1056/NEJMra1507771

Vowles, K. E., Witkiewitz, K., Levell, J., Sowden, G., & Ashworth, J. (2017). Are reductions in pain intensity and pain-related distress necessary? An analysis of within-treatment change trajectories in relation to improved functioning following interdisciplinary acceptance and commitment therapy for adults with chronic pain. *Journal of Consulting and Clinical Psychology, 85*, 87–98. http://dx.doi.org/10.1037/ccp0000159

Vranceanu, A. M., Jupiter, J. B., Mudgal, C. S., & Ring, D. (2010). Predictors of pain intensity and disability after minor hand surgery. *The Journal of Hand Surgery, 35*, 956–960. http://dx.doi.org/10.1016/j.jhsa.2010.02.001

Wang, D., & Teichtahl, H. (2007). Opioids, sleep architecture and sleep-disordered breathing. *Sleep Medicine Reviews, 11*, 35–46. http://dx.doi.org/10.1016/j.smrv.2006.03.006

Wang, D., Teichtahl, H., Drummer, O., Goodman, C., Cherry, G., Cunnington, D., & Kronborg, I. (2005). Central sleep apnea in stable methadone maintenance treatment patients. *Chest, 128*, 1348–1356. http://dx.doi.org/10.1378/chest.128.3.1348

Wang, D., Teichtahl, H., Goodman, C., Drummer, O., Grunstein, R. R., & Kronborg, I. (2008). Subjective daytime sleepiness and daytime function in patients on stable methadone maintenance treatment: Possible mechanisms. *Journal of Clinical Sleep Medicine, 4*, 557–562.

Webster, L. R., Choi, Y., Desai, H., Webster, L., & Grant, B. J. B. (2008). Sleep-disordered breathing and chronic opioid therapy. *Pain Medicine, 9*, 425–432. http://dx.doi.org/10.1111/j.1526-4637.2007.00343.x

Weingarten, T. N., Moeschler, S. M., Ptaszynski, A. E., Hooten, W. M., Beebe, T. J., & Warner, D. O. (2008). An assessment of the association between smoking status, pain intensity, and functional interference in patients with chronic pain. *Pain Physician, 11*, 643–653.

Wertli, M. M., Burgstaller, J. M., Weiser, S., Steurer, J., Kofmehl, R., & Held, U. (2014). Influence of catastrophizing on treatment outcome in patients with nonspecific low back pain: A systematic review. *Spine, 39*, 263–273. http://dx.doi.org/10.1097/BRS.0000000000000110

Wicksell, R. K., Kemani, M., Jensen, K., Kosek, E., Kadetoff, D., Sorjonen, K., . . . Olsson, G. L. (2013). Acceptance and commitment therapy for fibromyalgia: A randomized controlled trial. *European Journal of Pain, 17*, 599–611. http://dx.doi.org/10.1002/j.1532-2149.2012.00224.x

Williams, A. C., Eccleston, C., & Morley, S. (2012). Psychological therapies for the management of chronic pain (excluding headache) in adults. *Cochrane Database of Systematic Reviews, 11*. http://dx.doi.org/10.1002/14651858. CD007407.pub3

Wilson, A. C., Moss, A., Palermo, T. M., & Fales, J. L. (2014). Parent pain and catastrophizing are associated with pain, somatic symptoms, and pain-related disability among early adolescents. *Journal of Pediatric Psychology, 39*, 418–426. http://dx.doi.org/10.1093/jpepsy/jst094

Witvrouw, E., Pattyn, E., Almqvist, K. F., Crombez, G., Accoe, C., Cambier, D., & Verdonk, R. (2009). Catastrophic thinking about pain as a predictor of length of hospital stay after total knee arthroplasty: A prospective study. *Knee Surgery, Sports Traumatology, Arthroscopy, 17*, 1189–1194. http://dx.doi.org/10.1007/s00167-009-0817-x

Woods, M. P., & Asmundson, G. J. (2008). Evaluating the efficacy of graded in vivo exposure for the treatment of fear in patients with chronic back pain: A randomized controlled clinical trial. *Pain, 136*, 271–280. http://dx.doi.org/10.1016/j.pain.2007.06.037

Yoshino, A., Okamoto, Y., Okada, G., Takamura, M., Ichikawa, N., Shibasaki, C., . . . Yamawaki, S. (2018). Changes in resting-state brain networks after cognitive–behavioral therapy for chronic pain. *Psychological Medicine, 48*, 1148–1156. http://dx.doi.org/10.1017/S0033291717002598

Youngstedt, S. D., Kline, C. E., Elliott, J. A., Zielinski, M. R., Devlin, T. M., & Moore, T. A. (2016). Circadian phase-shifting effects of bright light, exercise, and bright light + exercise. *Journal of Circadian Rhythms, 14*, 2. http://dx.doi.org/10.5334/jcr.137

Zeidan, F., Martucci, K. T., Kraft, R. A., Gordon, N. S., McHaffie, J. G., & Coghill, R. C. (2011). Brain mechanisms supporting the modulation of pain by mindfulness meditation. *The Journal of Neuroscience, 31*, 5540–5548. http://dx.doi.org/10.1523/JNEUROSCI.5791-10.2011

Index

About the Author

Beth D. Darnall, PhD, is clinical professor in the Department of Anesthesiology, Perioperative and Pain Medicine, and by courtesy, Psychiatry and Behavioral Sciences, at Stanford University. She is principal investigator for multiple national pain and opioid reduction research projects that test the efficacy and mechanisms of psychological treatments in individuals with acute and chronic pain. She investigates mechanisms of pain catastrophizing, targeted pain psychology treatments she has developed, online perioperative behavioral treatments she has developed to reduce postsurgical pain and opioid use, and patient-centered opioid tapering for community outpatients. She delivers pain psychology and opioid reduction lectures and workshops nationally and internationally. She received a presidential commendation from the American Academy of Pain Medicine and currently serves as cochair of their Behavioral Medicine Committee.

She is author of *The Opioid-Free Pain Relief Kit* (2016) and *Less Pain, Fewer Pills: Avoid the Dangers of Prescription Opioids and Gain Control Over Chronic Pain* (2014), and coauthor of the American Pain Society book *Principles of Analgesic Use* (2016, 7th ed.). She spoke at the 2018 World Economic Forum (Davos, Switzerland) on the psychology of pain relief, and has been featured in major media outlets, including *O* magazine, *Forbes*, *Scientific American*, *The Washington Post*, BBC Radio, *Nature*, and *Time* magazine.

Website: bethdarnall.com
Twitter: @bethdarnall

About the Series Editor

Ellen A. Dornelas, PhD, is the director for cancer clinical research at Hartford Healthcare Cancer Institute in Connecticut and associate professor of clinical medicine at the University of Connecticut School of Medicine. Dr. Dornelas received her degree in health psychology from Ferkauf Graduate School of Psychology, Yeshiva University, New York, NY. She has focused her career on the integration of practice and research in clinical health psychology. Dr. Dornelas is recognized for her expertise in treating people with heart disease as well as cancer. She has supervised and mentored students for over two decades. Dr. Dornelas has authored multiple books and journal articles and is a featured guest expert on APA's Psychotherapy Video Series. She is a Fellow in American Psychological Association's Division 29 (Society for the Advancement of Psychotherapy) and a practicing psychotherapist.